COVID-19 and the Heart
A Case-Based Pocket Guide

T0175987

NOTICE

Medicine is an ever-changing science. As new research and clinical experience broaden our knowledge, changes in treatment and drug therapy are required. The authors and the publisher of this work have checked with sources believed to be reliable in their efforts to provide information that is complete and generally in accord with the standards accepted at the time of publication. However, in view of the possibility of human error or changes in medical sciences, neither the authors nor the publisher nor any other party who has been involved in the preparation or publication of this work warrants that the information contained herein is in every respect accurate or complete, and they disclaim all responsibility for any errors or omissions or for the results obtained from use of the information contained in this work. Readers are encouraged to confirm the information contained herein with other sources. For example and in particular, readers are advised to check the product information sheet included in the package of each drug they plan to administer to be certain that the information contained in this work is accurate and that changes have not been made in the recommended dose or in the contraindications for administration. This recommendation is of particular importance in connection with new or infrequently used drugs.

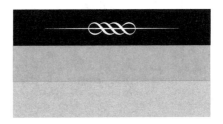

COVID-19 and the Heart
A Case-Based Pocket Guide

Muhammad Saad, MD
Department of Cardiology
Mount Sinai Morningside/BronxCare Hospital
New York

Timothy J. Vittorio, MS, MD
Department of Cardiology
BronxCare Hospital Center
Bronx, New York

New York Chicago San Francisco Athens London Madrid Mexico City
Milan New Delhi Singapore Sydney Toronto

COVID-19 and the Heart: A Case-Based Pocket Guide

1 2 3 4 5 6 7 8 9   LCR   26 25 24 23 22 21

ISBN 978-1-264-26670-8
MHID 1-264-26670-7

This book was set in Palatino LT Std by KnowledgeWorks Global Ltd.
The editors were Andrew Moyer, Jason Malley, and Kim J. Davis.
The production supervisor was Richard Ruzycka.
Project management was provided by Nitesh Sharma, KnowledgeWorks Global Ltd.
The cover designer was W2 Design.

This book is printed on acid-free paper.

Library of Congress Cataloging-in-Publication Data

Names: Saad, Muhammad, MD, editor. | Vittorio, Timothy J., editor.
Title: COVID-19 and the heart : a case-based pocket guide / [edited by] Muhammad Saad, Timothy J. Vittorio.
Description: New York : McGraw-Hill Education, [2022] | Includes bibliographical references and index. | Summary: "Everything you need to know to date about COVID-19 and how it affects the heart"—Provided by publisher.
Identifiers: LCCN 2021021202 (print) | LCCN 2021021203 (ebook) | ISBN 9781264266708 (paperback ; alk. paper) | ISBN 1264266707 (paperback ; alk. paper) | ISBN 9781264266715 (ebook) | ISBN 1264266715 (ebook)
Subjects: MESH: COVID-19—complications | Cardiovascular Diseases—complications | Case Reports | Handbook
Classification: LCC RA644.C67 (print) | LCC RA644.C67 (ebook) | NLM WC 39 | DDC 616.2/414—dc23
LC record available at https://lccn.loc.gov/2021021202
LC ebook record available at https://lccn.loc.gov/2021021203

McGraw Hill Education books are available at special quantity discounts to use as premiums and sales promotions or for use in corporate training programs. To contact a representative, please visit the Contact Us pages at www.mhprofessional.com.

To my parents (Saeeda Azhar and Azhar Hussain), for all the care and love you have provided to us. To my wife (Wajiha Saad) and daughters (Zariyah Saad and Fabiha Saad) for creating peaceful environment for me to prosper. To all my siblings (Fareeha, Ashar, and Anas) for always supporting me. Finally, to all my mentors, colleagues and juniors for a great inspiration to me, thank you all.

MUHAMMAD SAAD

I dedicate this book to my family for their constant support, encouragement, patience, and love. Thank you as well to my mentors, teachers, and colleagues, for shaping my medical education and making me the physician I am today. Most of all, I dedicate this book to the patients who have entrusted me with their care.

TIMOTHY J. VITTORIO

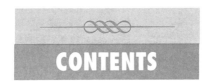

CONTENTS

CONTRIBUTORS

Fareeha Alavi
Department of Internal Medicine
BronxCare Hospital Center
Bronx, New York
8. COVID-19 and Hypertension

Nisha Ali, MD
Department of Internal Medicine
BronxCare Health System
Bronx, New York
2. COVID-19 and Acute Coronary Syndrome (ACS)

Shoaib Ashraf
Department of Internal Medicine
BronxCare Hospital Center
Bronx, New York
1. Introduction to COVID-19 and Cardiovascular Disease

Angel De La Cruz, MD
Department of Internal Medicine
BronxCare Hospital Center
Bronx, New York
9. COVID-19 and Cardiogenic Shock

Miguel Rodriguez Guerra
Department of Internal Medicine
BronxCare Hospital Center
Bronx, New York
4. COVID-19 and Heart Failure

Muhammad K. Guhjjar, MD
Department of Medicine
BronxCare Hospital Center
Bronx, New York
4. COVID-19 and Heart Failure

Hitesh Gurjar, MD
Department of Internal Medicine
BronxCare Hospital Center
Bronx, New York
8. COVID-19 and Hypertension

Muhammad Hassan, BS
Department of Cardiology
BronxCare Hospital Center
Bronx, New York
10. COVID-19 Management Strategies

Wajiha Jahangir
Department of Internal Medicine
BronxCare Hospital Center
Bronx, New York
2. COVID-19 and Acute Coronary Syndrome (ACS)

Sarthak Kulshreshtha, Medical Student
Department of Internal Medicine
BronxCare Hospital Center
Bronx, New York
10. COVID-19 Management Strategies

Niel Shah, MD
Department of Internal Medicine
BronxCare Hospital Center
Bronx, New York
1. Introduction to COVID-19 and Cardiovascular Disease
7. COVID-19 and Myopericardial Disease

Nikee Shrestha, MD
Department of Internal Medicine
BronxCare Hospital Center
Bronx, New York
1. Introduction to COVID-19 and Cardiovascular Disease

Saaria Shoaib
Department of Internal Medicine
BronxCare Hospital Center
Bronx, New York
1. Introduction to COVID-19 and Cardiovascular Disease

Rishi Shrivastav, MD
Fellow in Cardiovascular Medicine
Icahn School of Medicine at Mount Sinai Morningside
New York, New York
6. COVID-19 and Valvular Heart Disease

Amandeep Singh, MD
Division of Cardiology
BronxCare Hospital Center
Bronx, New York
6. COVID-19 and Valvular Heart Disease
9. COVID-19 and Cardiogenic Shock

Jeirym Miranda Tejada
Department of Internal Medicine
BronxCare Hospital Center
Bronx, New York
5. COVID-19 and Cardiac Arrythmias

Timothy J. Vittorio, MS, MD
Department of Cardiology
BronxCare Hospital Center
Bronx, New York
5. COVID-19 and Cardiac Arrythmias
7. COVID-19 and Myopericardial Disease

Maleeha Zahid, MD
Department of Internal Medicine
BronxCare Hospital Center
Bronx, NY
3. COVID-19 and Thromboembolism

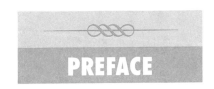

PREFACE

Presently, the world is faced with the most challenging pandemic of the modern era, that of severe acute respiratory syndrome 2 (SARS-CoV-2) infection which causes coronavirus disease (COVID-19). This first edition of our textbook *COVID-19 and the Heart: A Case-Based Pocket Guide* was developed as a unique and practical means to assist healthcare workers actively engaged in this ongoing pandemic. We constructed the text as user friendly as possible by utilizing a personal conversation style of writing.

This book is essentially a user's manual to guide the medical practitioner in making adequate clinical judgement quickly with respect to the cardiac manifestations of COVID-19 disease. The book is divided into chapters based on genuine clinical cases with a proposed approach for each case.

To help orient and to prevent excessive details to the reader, we added several key points at the end of each case complementing and highlighting the major points throughout the clinical content with the intention of allowing an easier and quicker review.

It is our goal that this book will serve as an effective teaching tool in the recognition and management of the cardiac sequelae due to COVID-19 disease.

We hope that you enjoy this book and find it useful.

Muhammad Saad, MD
Timothy J. Vittorio, MS, MD

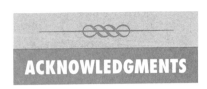

ACKNOWLEDGMENTS

This book would not be possible without the input and support of many individuals, specifically the cardiology fellows and internal medicine residents who assisted us in writing the individual chapters.

We would like to extend our gratitude to Dr. Sridhar Chilimuri, an indefatigable leader, who has provided inestimable guidance to the Department of Medicine throughout the pandemic.

As with all of our endeavors, this book would also have been impossible without the support of our families, to whom we are always indebted.

COVID-19 and the Heart
A Case-Based Pocket Guide

CHAPTER 1

Introduction to COVID-19 and Cardiovascular Disease

NIKEE SHRESTHA, NIEL SHAH,
SHOAIB ASHRAF, SAARIA SHOAIB

CASE PRESENTATION

A female patient in her late forties presented to the emergency department with neck swelling and pain on the right side for the last week. She had a significant past medical history of noninsulin-dependent diabetes mellitus, hypertension, morbid obesity, and iron deficiency anemia. The patient had a right internal jugular (IJ) tunneled catheter for iron infusions. She reported having a headache and myalgia 2 weeks prior, which she thought was the regular flu, and symptoms improved without any treatment. Her vital signs on admission were body temperature of 99.3°F, blood pressure of 139/77 mmHg, sinus tachycardia of 114 beats/min, respiratory rate of 17 breaths/min, and oxygen saturation of 98% on room air. Physical examination was unremarkable except right neck tenderness. A computed tomography (CT) scan of the neck and soft tissue with contrast showed the right IJ vein almost entirely thrombosed from its origin at the skull base to the right subclavian vein (Figure 1-1A). Meanwhile, CT scan of the chest showed diffuse ground-glass opacity within the lungs (Figure 1-1B). The right central vein subcutaneous port-a-cath access was removed, and she was begun on systemic anticoagulation with warfarin. Additional workup showed high factor VIII, D-dimer, low serum iron, and negative blood culture. The patient was suspected of having coronavirus disease 19 (COVID-19) as a cause of IJ thrombus. Anti-SARS-CoV-2 antibodies were done and reported positive.

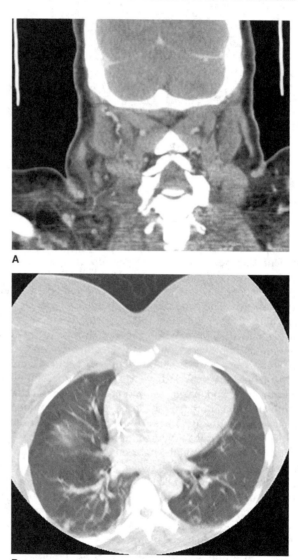

A

B

FIGURE 1-1 (A) Computed tomography (CT) scan of the neck and soft tissue with contrast showed the right internal jugular vein almost entirely thrombosed. **(B)** Diffuse ground-glass opacity within the lungs suggestive on CT scan of the chest.

PATHOGENESIS OF COVID-19

COVID-19 is a viral infection caused by SARS-CoV-2. This disease, which eventually progressed as a pandemic, was first reported in Wuhan, China, in December 2019. As of December 2020, 66.7 million cases were reported worldwide and the mortality was 1.53 million. The major cause of COVID-19–related mortality is severe acute respiratory distress syndrome (ARDS). However, it has also been observed that COVID-19 affects all major organ systems, including the cardiovascular system. The long-term implication of COVID-19–related cardiovascular involvement is still unknown.

SARS-CoV-2: SARS-CoV-2 is a single-stranded, enveloped RNA virus. It belongs to the genus *betacoronavirus*, which is similar to the two pathogenic coronaviruses known to humankind: severe acute respiratory syndrome coronavirus (SARS-CoV) and Middle East respiratory syndrome coronavirus (MERS-CoV). Phylogenetic analysis showed that SARS-CoV-2 is closely related to bat-derived coronavirus of the genus *betacoronavirus* (about 88%), SARS-CoV (about 79%), and MERS-CoV (about 50%). Additionally, SARS-CoV and SARS-CoV-2 both use angiotensin-converting enzyme 2 (ACE2) as an attachment receptor to bind to the host cell, implying similarity in the biological features between them.

SARS-CoV-2 comprises four structural proteins: spike protein (S), envelope (E), membrane (M), and nucleocapsid (N). The S protein is responsible for binding to the receptor-binding domain of the ACE2 receptor of host cell, which facilitates entry into the host cell. ACE2 is found in abundance in respiratory tract epithelial cells, cardiac myocytes, and vascular endothelial cells. After binding to the cellular receptor, transmembrane serine protease (TMPRSS2) primes the cleavage of the S protein at the S1/S2 and the S2′ site. The S2 subunit then causes fusion of viral and cellular membranes and endocytosis into the cells, releasing the viral genome into the cytoplasm. Viral genome then replicates, structural proteins are translated, and numerous viral particles are assembled and released through exocytosis. In this process SARS-CoV-2 internalizes ACE2 from the cell surface, downregulating its expression. Another pathway of entry in the host cell is through the endosomal entry pathway, which might be the major entry pathway for coronaviruses for infection in vitro, but its importance in vivo is unclear.

Role of ACE2: ACE2 is one of the major components of the renin-angiotensin-aldosterone system (RAAS). It is a peptidase enzyme that acts on angiotensin II and converts it into the cardioprotective peptide angiotensin. Angiotensin II is known to cause vasoconstriction, retention of sodium via aldosterone, inflammation, and fibrosis. Angiotensin, on the other hand, is known to be cardioprotective due to its vasodilatory, antiproliferative, anti-inflammatory, and antifibrotic properties. Because SARS-CoV-2 causes internalization of ACE2 receptors and reduces its availability on its surface, there is increased action of angiotensin II and decreased action of angiotensin promoting vasoconstriction, inflammation, and fibrosis. Initially, there was some concern of increased risk of COVID-19 infection in patients on medications acting on the RAAS, which was later confuted. In fact, studies have shown that RAAS blockade increases ACE2 expression/activity.

Immunosuppression and Hyperinflammation (Cytokine Storm): Pathogenesis of COVID-19 infection involves the immune system to a greater extent. It has been reported that severe COVID-19 infection affects different immunological pathways to cause immune deficiency. SARS-CoV-2 has been found to cause lymphopenia, with a decrease in both CD4$^+$ and CD8$^+$ cells. Furthermore, there is evidence of T-cell PD1 and TIM3 overexpression, which is suggestive of T-cell exhaustion. Several studies have demonstrated a positive correlation between lymphopenia, T-cell exhaustion, and elevated levels of interleukin (IL)-6, IL-10, and tumor necrosis factor (TNF)-α. All of these can cause immunosuppression and allow the virus to evade the immune system. SARS-CoV-1 and MERS use double-membrane vesicles, which lack pattern recognition receptors (PRRs). They also interfere with antigen presentation by major histocompatibility complex (MHC) and hence T-cell activation.

Generally, virus infection in the host cell activates the innate immune system, resulting in natural killer (NK) cell–mediated cell lysis. Adaptive immune system activation causes cytotoxic

CD8$^+$ cell–mediated lysis of virus-infected cells. After viral clearance, the antigen-presenting cells and CD8$^+$ cells undergo apoptosis to limit further immune activation. However, there is an unchecked activation of the innate immune system caused by lymphopenia and T-cell exhaustion during the mentioned process resulting in the production of proinflammatory cytokines in an unrestrained way, which is known as a cytokine storm. Cytokines such as IL-1, IL-6, IL-18, interferon (IFN)-γ, and TNF-α have been found in cases with severe COVID-19 infection. Production of inflammatory cytokines in COVID-19 has been linked to severe disease and multiorgan failure. Inflammatory markers such as erythrocyte sedimentation rate (ESR), C-reactive protein (CRP), ferritin, and lactate dehydrogenase (LDH) can be used as indicators of disease severity (Figure 1-2).

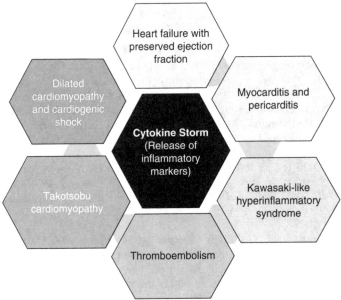

FIGURE 1-2 **Cytokine storm manifestation in the cardiovascular system.**

VARIOUS STRAINS OF COVID-19

Coronavirus has mutated to produce various strains that have been found globally. One of the most prominent infectious strains, referred to as "SARS-CoV-2 VOC 202012/01" or "B.1.1.7," has been recently described in the United Kingdom. This strain has a mutation in the S protein that binds tightly to the ACE2 receptor. This strain has not been associated with severe illness or higher mortality thus far. More research is ongoing to evaluate the pathogenicity of various strains worldwide. Recently, South Africa announced the emergence of a new strain independent of the UK strains. SARS-CoV-2 Sequencing for Public Health Emergency Response, Epidemiology, and Surveillance (SPHERES) is a national genomics initiative led by the Centers for Disease Control and Prevention (CDC) to monitor and coordinate COVID-19 evolution and spread and guide diagnostic and therapeutic targets.

RELATIONSHIP BETWEEN COVID-19 AND CARDIOVASCULAR DIEASES

Cardiovascular Diseases as a Risk for COVID-19 Infection: Since the beginning of the COVID-19 pandemic in Wuhan, China, many studies and case reports have shown adverse outcomes related to COVID-19 in patients with preexisting cardiovascular diseases such as hypertension, coronary artery disease (CAD), and heart failure (HF). Furthermore, the occurrence of severe disease requiring critical care management and mortality is also reported to be higher in individuals with such comorbidities. In a meta-analysis of 6 studies with 1527 patients, the prevalence of hypertension, cardio-cerebrovascular diseases, and diabetes in patients with COVID-19 were 17.1%, 16.4%, and 9.7%, respectively, with high critical care unit admissions (Table 1-1).

Prevention of COVID-19 Infection in Cardiovascular Disease: Preexisting cardiovascular disease has been associated with severe COVID-19 illness and poor outcomes. Hence, it is important to make all efforts to prevent transmission of the virus. Exposure to infected people should be minimized as much as possible. Since hospital-associated transmission is a possibility, hospital visits should be kept

TABLE 1-1 Pathogenesis of Cardiovascular Disease in COVID-19 Infection

S.N.	Cardiovascular Effects	Incidence	Pathogenesis
1.	Arrhythmia	17% in ICU patients	• Hypoxia due to ARDS • Angiotensin II–mediated electrolyte disturbances • Systemic hyperinflammation affecting cardiac ion channels • Drug effect (hydroxychloroquine, chloroquine, antivirals)
2.	Myocardial injury: myocarditis, heart failure, cardiogenic shock	7%-20%	• Cytokine–mediated release of ROS, NO, and superoxide ion–mediated injury • Systemic hyperinflammation–mediated apoptosis of cardiac cells • Direct myocardial cytotoxicity by SARS-CoV-2 • Hypoxia–mediated myocardial damage • Hyperinflammation and catecholamine surge due to stress causing stress cardiomyopathy • ARDS causing pulmonary HTN and right heart failure
3.	Acute coronary syndrome	2%-4%	• Systemic inflammation, microthrombi formation resulting in endothelial damage and plaque rupture • Microvascular dysfunction caused by direct cytotoxicity of SARS-CoV-2 in pericytes of coronary arteries
4.	Hypertension	17%	• Angiotensin II–mediated vasoconstriction, sodium and water retention, inflammation, fibrosis • Reduced activity of angiotensin, which is anti-inflammatory, antifibrotic, and vasodilatory

(Continued)

TABLE 1-1 Pathogenesis of Cardiovascular Disease in COVID-19 Infection *(Continued)*

S.N.	Cardiovascular Effects	Incidence	Pathogenesis
5.	Thromboembolism	27% (ICU)	• Cytokine–mediated damage of endothelial cell-activating coagulation cascade
		6% (in wards)	• Angiotensin II–mediated vascular inflammation
			• Prolonged immobility in critical cases
			• Reduced thrombolysis due to hyperinflammation
6.	Valvular damage	Rare	• Angiotensin II–mediated inflammation and fibrosis
7.	Pericardial disease	Unknown	• Angiotensin II–mediated serosal inflammation and fibrosis

ARDS, acute respiratory distress syndrome; HTN, hypertension; ICU, intensive care unit; NO, nitric oxide; ROS, reactive oxygen species; SARS-CoV-2, severe acute respiratory syndrome coronavirus 2.

to a minimum and when necessary, inpatient stay duration should be as short as possible.

Chronic cardiovascular conditions that require outpatient monitoring or follow-up should be managed by telemedicine. Additionally, the use of remote monitoring devices such as pulmonary artery pressure sensors and CardioMEMS should be considered. All the standard precautions should be taken for patients with acute cardiac disease or those requiring a hospital visit or admission. Furthermore, they should be managed in a COVID-free zone of the hospital if possible, proper hygiene precautions should be adopted, and all the healthcare workers should be donned in appropriate personal protective equipment (PPE). Elective procedures should be kept to a minimum during the COVID surge to decrease transmission and avoid overloading the health system. Nevertheless, patients should be educated to seek medical attention whenever required and instructed to practice safety precautions to avoid transmission.

Hemodynamic Monitoring in COVID-19: Cardiovascular sequelae in patients with COVID-19 such as myocarditis, shock, and coagulopathy, along with high positive end-expiratory pressure (PEEP) mechanical ventilation for ARDS, demand meticulous hemo-dynamic monitoring as patients are highly susceptible to end-organ hypoperfusion. Various noninvasive and invasive technologies can be used for monitoring of intravascular volume status.

Noninvasive techniques include echocardiography (transthoracic or transesophageal), and noninvasive cardiac monitoring (NICOM). Echocardiogram gives us valuable information regarding ventricu-lar function, size, and pressures as well as volume responsiveness by assessing inferior vena cava (IVC) diameter. However, it can only provide cross-sectional information, which makes it unsuitable for continuous monitoring. It also requires expert individuals and increases exposure of healthcare workers.

Minimally invasive techniques like pulse index contour car-diac output (PiCCO), lithium dilution cardiac output (LiDCO), and FloTrac devices can be used. Invasive techniques like pulmonary artery catheterization (PAC) can be used for continuous monitor-ing of intravascular volume status and cardiac function, but PAC can overestimate left ventricular volume in ARDS patients requir-ing high PEEP ventilation and carries risk for pulmonary artery perforation.

Cardiac Arrest Management in COVID-19: SARS-CoV-2, through its direct effect on the heart, causes myocardial dysfunction, which itself and/or in conjunction with ARDS contributes to cardiac arrhythmias and cardiac arrest. Management of cardiac arrest in COVID-19 follows the advanced cardiac life support (ACLS) proto-col with some modifications that emphasize preventing or limiting risk of aerosolization to healthcare workers. The number of individ-uals involved should be kept to a required minimum. All the health personnel involved in the cardiac arrest management should be donned in full PPE. For airway management, use of nonrebreather or face mask with high-flow oxygen and insertion of oral airway is recommended for oxygenation until additional help arrives for car-diopulmonary resuscitation (CPR). Also, a bag valve mask attached to a high-efficiency particulate absorbing (HEPA) filter can be used while ensuring a tight seal with the face mask. Video laryngoscopy should be preferred over direct laryngoscopy for intubation and chest compressions should be held during intubation, which help in minimizing the risk of aerosol transmission to the person performing intubation. The patient should be attached to a ventilator with a HEPA filter attached and the ventilator closed circuit should be ensured to prevent leakage of aerosol to the environment. Intraosseous (IO) access should be considered whenever a peripheral or central intravenous (IV) line is difficult because it is faster, minimizing the exposure time. Mechanical CPR devices should be used whenever available. Defibrillation, being a non–aerosol-generating procedure, is recommended early in the case of shockable rhythm, which will shorten the duration of resuscitation and minimize exposure time.

Management of COVID-19 in Patients with LVAD or Heart Transplant: Patients with left ventricular assist device (LVAD) or HF are considered a vulnerable population for severe COVID-19 given their high cardiovascular risk, risk for infection, and thrombosis; thus extra precautions are required to prevent transmission of SARS-CoV-2. Whenever possible, remote monitoring of LVAD should be preferred. Thromboembolic predisposition in COVID-19 increases the risk of pump thrombosis in LVAD recipients, so therapeutic anticoagulation should be ensured in those patients. As discussed previously, hyperinflammation and cytokine storm plays a major role in the pathogenesis of COVID-19-related cardiovascular diseases and use of an LVAD is believed to be associated with an overall improved inflammatory profile in the setting of COVID-19.

Patients with a heart transplant have been reported to be infected with COVID-19. An early study in China involving 87 heart transplant patients reported that the patients who used extra precautionary measures to avoid exposure did not have a high rate of infection. Similarly, a multicenter survey from Germany involving 21 heart transplant patients with COVID-19 reported clinical presentation similar to nontransplant patients with 8 of 21 patients developing severe disease. However, mortality was found to be elevated in patients with severe disease (87.5%). Right ventricular dysfunction, arrhythmias, and thromboembolic events were seen in a group with severe disease compared with the nonsevere disease group.

Heart transplant patients are on high-dose immunosuppression, but the effect of immunosuppression on the disease course is unclear. It is believed to be obscuring the typical manifestations of COVID and may even confuse lab findings due to preexisting lymphopenia. Management initially is supportive, and several protocols have been used by transplant centers in terms of immunosuppressants, such as pausing mycophenolate mofetil, switching sirolimus to tacrolimus, and using high-dose corticosteroids. Due to the high mortality of heart transplant patients with COVID-19, utmost importance should be given to preventive measures. (1-5)

KEY POINTS

- Cytokine storm activated by COVID-19 can lead to myocardial fibrosis and endothelial damage.
- COVID-19 has been associated with worse outcomes in cardio-vascular disease patients.
- Telemedicine and remote monitoring should be performed in patients with cardiac conditions such as HF.

PATIENT EDUCATION

- All patients with a cardiac condition should be advised to wear a face mask and follow social distancing.
- Patients should be educated to seek medical attention whenever red flag symptoms are noticed.
- Red flag symptoms include shortness of breath, dizziness, myalgias, and body aches.

References

1. Zhou P, Yang X-L, Wang X-G, et al. A pneumonia outbreak associated with a new coronavirus of probable bat origin. *Nature*. 2020;579(7798):270-273.
2. Nishiga M, Wang DW, Han Y, Lewis DB, Wu JC. COVID-19 and cardio-vascular disease: from basic mechanisms to clinical perspectives. *Nat Rev Cardiol*. 2020;17(9):543-558.
3. Lu R, Zhao X, Li J, et al. Genomic characterisation and epidemiology of 2019 novel coronavirus: implications for virus origins and receptor binding. *Lancet Lond Engl*. 2020;395(10224):565-574.

4. Hoffmann M, Kleine-Weber H, Schroeder S, et al. SARS-CoV-2 cell entry depends on ACE2 and TMPRSS2 and is blocked by a clinically proven protease inhibitor. *Cell*. 2020;181(2):271-280.e8.
5. Sattar Y, Ullah W, Rauf H, et al. COVID-19 cardiovascular epidemiology, cellular pathogenesis, clinical manifestations and management. *Int J Cardiol Heart Vasc*. 2020;29:100589.

CHAPTER 2

COVID-19 and Acute Coronary Syndrome (ACS)

Nisha Ali, Wajiha Jahangir

CASE PRESENTATION

A 68-year-old male presented to the hospital for chest pain and shortness of breath (SOB). His medical history includes hypertension, type 2 diabetes mellitus, and hyperlipidemia. He is an active smoker, smoking 1 pack per day for the last 45 years. Family history is significant for a father with hypertension and coronary artery disease (CAD) in his 60s and mother with hypertension and diabetes mellitus.

The patient reports a 3-day history of worsening substernal chest pain radiating to the left shoulder. Pain was initially 4/10 in intensity, which later increased to 9/10. Chest pain was nonexertional and associated with SOB, nausea, and diaphoresis. No history of similar complaints in the past. One week prior to presentation, the patient reported low-grade fever, weakness, and loss of sense of taste. He was tested for COVID-19, which came back positive. Given the mild symptoms, he was advised to self-isolate at home and was prescribed azithromycin 500 mg for 5 days. He was advised to monitor his temperature at home and to seek medical attention if his symptoms persist or worsen. His symptoms improved except for loss of sense of taste.

En route to the hospital the patient received aspirin 320 mg orally by emergency medical services (EMS). In the emergency room he was tachycardic (heart rate [HR] 116 beats/min), blood pressure (BP) 168/95 mmHg, temperature 98.5°F, and oxygen saturation of

96% on room air. Electrocardiogram (ECG) showed ST elevation in the inferior leads with reciprocal changes in the anterolateral leads. He underwent coronary angiography with percutaneous coronary intervention (PCI) and drug-eluting stents placed in the right coronary artery. He was moved to the cardiac care unit and COVID testing was performed, which came back negative. COVID antibodies were positive. Transthoracic echocardiogram showed ejection fraction (EF) of 55%, grade 2 diastolic dysfunction, akinesia of the inferior wall, and pulmonary artery pressure of 48 mmHg. Laboratory data revealed elevated inflammatory marker, peaked cardiac troponin of 820 (normal <5), and pro-brain natriuretic peptide (BNP) of 1200 ng/L. The patient had an uncomplicated hospital stay and was discharged after 4 days.

INTRODUCTION

Epidemiology: According to a survey from China, 10%-25% of cases of COVID-19 infection had underlying CAD. It is associated with an extremely high mortality rate in CAD patients. In a hospital-wide observational study in the United Kingdom, hospital admissions for ACS have gone down by 40% (compared with 2019) from January to April 2020, and were partially recovered in May. Similarly, the rate of PCI declined by 21% in patients with ST elevation myocardial infarction (STEMI) partly because of fear of contracting COVID-19 infection in the hospital along with loss of healthcare benefits. Pain perception is also altered due to COVID–related neurologic involvement.

Pathophysiology: COVID-19 can create an inflammatory milieu, which can trigger thrombotic events such as ACS. Myocardial injury due to COVID-19 infection can manifest in myriad of clinical presentations. Plaque rupture, microembolism, and vasospasm are underlying mechanisms of COVID–induced myocardial injury. These abnormalities occur due to shear forces in the coronary circulation leading to vessel injury. Type 2 MI due to metabolic derangements and hypoxia can also present as ACS. Microvascular dysfunction due to cellular injury can also present with angina symptoms (Figure 2-1).

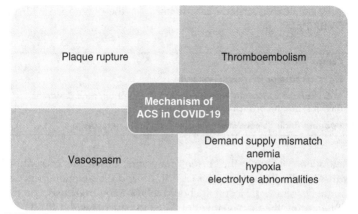

FIGURE 2-1 **Mechanism of myocardial infarction in COVID-19 infection.** ACS, acute coronary syndrome.

Presentation: Symptoms of MI in COVID-19 infection includes anginal chest pain and SOB along with typical features of viral pneumonia. Occasionally, ACS presentation is masked by respiratory symptoms; therefore, careful monitoring is required for timely diagnosis. Atypical presentations include syncope, dizziness, nausea, and fatigue.

ACS includes STEMI, non-ST elevation MI (NSTEMI), and unstable angina. MI can be classified into two types as per the fourth universal definition of MI:

- Type 1: Caused by plaque rupture or erosion
- Type II: Caused by oxygen supply and demand mismatch

The majority of MI cases in COVID-19 are attributed to demand and supply mismatch and a few are related to plaque rupture.

Diagnostic modality: Although clinical history is the cornerstone of diagnosis, some patients can have overlapping symptoms between COVID-19 sepsis and ACS. Elevated troponin also can be seen in other COVID–related thromboembolic disorders.

The following criteria can be used for the diagnosis of MI in COVID-19:

- **Clinical features of MI**
- **Elevated cardiac markers (troponin)**
- **ECG changes consistent with ischemia (ST elevation, new Q waves, new left bundle branch block [LBBB])**
- **Imaging findings consistent new loss of viable myocardium**

Management: Due to the current pandemic, all patients presenting with ACS should be tested for COVID-19 and the isolation protocol should be followed. Hospitals should follow a comprehensive protocol regarding the management of ACSs in patients with COVID-19. All patients should wear a mask and all staff should wear personal protective equipment (PPE). (1-6)

- Approach to STEMI: Early diagnosis and intervention are the key regardless of COVID-19. All patients with STEMI should be treated with standard aspirin, $P2Y_{12}$ inhibitor, and anticoagulation.
- Prehospital care: In case of STEMI, EMS should alert the nearest PCI centers. Clinical information, ECG, and detailed COVID-19 exposure history should be provided. In case of NTSEMI, COVID-19 nasopharyngeal swabs should be sent before admission to the cardiology unit.
- Hospital care: STEMI with COVID-19 infection should be transferred to the catheterization laboratory with standard PPE, surgical mask, gown, and gloves. Vital signs, oxygen saturation, and nasopharyngeal swabs should be promptly conducted. After angiography, the patient should be transferred to the COVID unit and the Cath Lab should be terminally cleaned. Air exchange timings in the Cath Lab should be maintained at 15 exchanges per hour.

In case of STEMI with cardiac arrest, intubation and resuscitation should be performed with full precautions along with powered air-purifying respirator before angiography is performed.

Thrombolytics can be administered alternatively based on hospital protocol if PCI is not available. Risk of COVID–associated thromboembolism and disseminated intravascular coagulation should be considered before fibrinolytics. Factors such as patient's comorbidities, hemodynamic stability, age, severity of the disease, patients' prognosis, and hospital resource limitation should also be considered.

PCI should also be considered over coronary artery bypass graft (CABG) in COVID-19 patients. Patients should be referred to COVID-free surgery centers after complete evaluation by nasal swabs and computed tomography (CT) scans (Figure 2-2).

- Approach to NSTEMI and unstable angina: Patients with high-risk NSTEMI should undergo immediate invasive revascularization. On the other hand, patients with low- to intermediate-risk NSTEMI and unstable angina can be treated conservatively with aspirin, $P2Y_{12}$ inhibitor, and anticoagulation. PCI is reserved

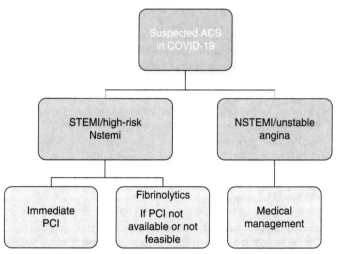

FIGURE 2-2 Management algorithm of ACS in COVID-19 infection. NSTEMI, non-ST elevation myocardial infarction; PCI, percutaneous coronary intervention; STEMI, ST elevation myocardial infarction.

for patients who remain unstable or have ongoing evidence of myocardial ischemia. All patients with NSTEMI and COVID-19 infection should be treated in the COVID unit with telemetry support.

Complications of MI in COVID-19: Due to the delayed presentation of MI in the COVID-19 era, mechanical complications have been reported in the literature post MI. Free wall rupture, ventricular septal defect, and left ventricular aneurysms have been observed in post-MI patients with COIVID-19. Inotropic support and bedside placement of intra-aortic balloon pump (IABP) can be considered as a bridge to definitive surgical treatment.

Prognosis and monitoring: ACS in COVID-19 patients has been associated with worse prognosis along with higher morbidity and mortality. Patients should be monitored post discharge with frequent telehealth visits and medication optimization. Risk factor modifications should be advised to avoid future events.

KEY POINTS

- ACS in COVID-19 infection has been associated with higher morbidity and mortality.
- Mechanisms includes plaque rupture, vasospasm, and thromboembolic events.
- PCI should be considered in STEMI and high-risk NSTEMI patients with comprehensive precaution as per hospital protocol.

PATIENT EDUCATION

- MI (heart attack) presents with symptoms of chest pain, SOB, nausea, and fatigue.
- Immediate medical attention should be sought as MI is a medical emergency and can be associated with fatal outcomes.
- Precautions such as wearing mask can help prevent COVID-19, but physicians should always be consulted if symptoms are suggestive of MI.

References

1. Pinto DS. Coronavirus disease 2019 (COVID-19): myocardial infarction and other coronary artery disease issues. *UpToDate.* 2020.
2. Cevik M, Bamford CGG, Ho A. COVID-19 pandemic-a focused review for clinicians. *Clin Microbiol Infect.* 2020;26:842-847.
3. Liu Y, Li J, Feng Y. Critical care response to a hospital outbreak of the 2019-nCoV infection in Shenzhen, China. *Crit Care.* 2020;24(1):56.
4. Libby P, Loscalzo J, Ridker PM, et al. Inflammation, immunity, and infection in atherothrombosis: JACC Review Topic of the Week. *J Am Coll Cardiol.* 2018;72:2071.
5. Mafham MM, Spata E, Goldacre R, et al. COVID-19 pandemic and admission rates for and management of acute coronary syndromes in England. *Lancet.* 2020;396(10248):381-389.
6. Wang D, Hu B, Hu C, et al. Clinical characteristics of 138 hospitalized patients with 2019 novel coronavirus–infected pneumonia in Wuhan, China. *JAMA.* 2020;323(11):1061-1069.

CHAPTER 3

COVID-19 and Thromboembolism

Maleeha Zahid

CASE PRESENTATION

A 35-year-old male patient with a medical history of well-controlled hypertension and diabetes mellitus presented to the emergency room with left sided weakness when he woke up from sleep that progressed to paralysis of the left side of his body. The symptoms started 12 hours prior to his arrival. The patient also reported feeling shortness of breath for the last few days. He denied any recent sick contact, headache, photophobia, recreational drug use, and family history of note. His medications included metformin and hydrochlorothiazide. Vitals signs were temperature 97.6°F, blood pressure 153/117 mmHg, heart rate of 117 beats/min, and oxygen saturation of 91% on nonrebreather mask. His finger stick glucose was 98 mg/dl. Physical examination revealed alert, oriented male in mild respiratory distress. Pupillary examination revealed anisocoria. Lungs were clear to auscultation except bibasilar crackles, and heart sounds were normal. On neurological examination, the patient had hemiplegia of the left side of the body but had good strength on the right side of the body. Abdomen was soft without any organomegaly. Initial labs revealed mild leukocytosis (white blood cell [WBC] of 11.0 k/μl), with normal hemoglobin, electrolytes, and renal function. D-dimers were elevated at 1088 ng/ml. His initial international normalized ratio (INR) was 1.06, prothrombin time (PT) was 12.5 seconds, and partial thromboplastin time (PTT) was 30.7 seconds. He was also noted to have an elevated lactate dehydrogenase (LDH) level at 254 unit/L and elevated C-reactive protein at 17.2 mg/L. The patient tested positive for SARS-CoV-2 RNA via polymerase chain reaction testing. Chest X-ray revealed bilateral pulmonary opacities. Computed tomography (CT) of the head showed no evidence of acute intracranial hemorrhage or injury. CT angiogram of the brain revealed abrupt occlusion of the right M2 middle cerebral artery (MCA) inferior branch with lack of visible perfusion in the posterior inferior right MCA territory. Subsequent CT head showed interval development of a large acute right MCA distribution territorial infarct, with findings suspicious for thrombus involving a branch of the right M2 segment. The patient was diagnosed with acute right MCA stroke in the setting of COVID-19 infection. Since he was not a candidate for tissue plasminogen activator (tPA) due to the late presentation, he was given aspirin and high-intensity statin. He also received conservative management for COVID-19 pneumonia. After 48 hours of stroke symptoms, he was initiated on low-molecular-weight heparin (LMWH) for venous thromboembolism (VTE) prophylaxis. His oxygenation and hemodynamic parameters started to improve. His D-dimer and LDH started to trend down. He was later discharged to rehabilitation center for physical therapy.

Epidemiology: According to observational data, the incidence of thromboembolic disorder such as pulmonary embolism (PE) in COVID-19 infection ranges from 1.5%-9%. (1-3) Similarly, the incidence of asymptomatic deep venous thrombosis (DVT) in hospitalized patients with COVID infection ranges from 18%-20%. (1-3) Cerebrovascular accident was observed in 1%-6% of the population with COVID infection. More younger patients (median age 58 years) developed thromboembolic events in COVID infection with male gender predisposition. (1-3)

Pathophysiology: SARS-CoV-2 virus enters the cell via angiotensin-converting 2 receptors, which are expressed on the vascular endothelial cells. Both in vitro and autopsy studies have shown evidence of the invasion of vasculature by the virus. Autopsy studies have demonstrated the presence of intracellular virus and severe endothelial injury in the form of endotheliitis and apoptotic bodies in the vascular architecture of many organs including lungs, kidneys, and intestines. Dysregulated and uncontrolled host responses lead to the release of inflammatory cytokines such as interleukin (IL)-1, IL-6,

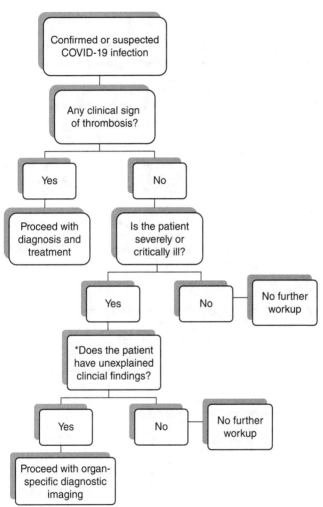

*Unexplained clinical findings in a COVID-19 patient include hypoxia out of proportion to the radiographic changes, signs of heart failure, lactic acidosis despite adequate resuscitation, cold extremities, new-onset limb or facial

FIGURE 3-1 Diagnostic algorithm of COVID-19–related thromboembolism.

IL-8, and tumor necrosis factor (TNF)-α. IL-6 is a major cytokine that is implicated in the pathogenesis of coagulopathy.(1) It triggers the activation of tissue factor expression and increased platelet and fibrinogen production. Tissue factor then triggers activation of factor Xa, factor VIIa, and thrombin production. These microthrombi are stabilized by neutrophils via release of neutrophil extracellular traps (NETs). Degradation of tissue factor antagonist by neutrophil elastases leads to further immobilization of these microthrombi.(2)

It is noteworthy that IL-6 levels are considerably higher in critically ill COVID-19 patients compared with similarly ill patients due to bacterial pneumonia. IL-1 and TNF-α have also been implicated in COVID-19–related coagulopathy due to their role in the suppression of endogenous anticoagulant pathways. In addition, SARS-CoV-2 also leads to disruption of the balance between the plasmin and urokinase pathway, which causes fibrin accumulation. Hypoxia is another significant symptom of COVID-19 infection and a potent stimulator of thrombosis. The resulting inflammatory cascade can lead to both microvascular and macrovascular thrombosis.

In addition to the inflammatory response, pathogens including SARS-CoV-2 can also lead to the activation of complement. Complement activation products have been detected on the circulating red blood cells in COVID-19 patients. As the illness progresses, dysregulation of the complement activation pathway can occur, which can further potentiate tissue damage. In patients with severe COVID-19 illness, overactivation of the complement pathways can also occur. Together with a prothrombotic state and cytokine release syndrome, overactivated complement cascade can lead to widespread organ damage and clinical deterioration of these patients.

Diagnostic Evaluation: Differentiating COVID-19–induced coagulopathy from disseminated intravascular coagulation (DIC) often can be challenging. Significant elevations in D-dimers can be seen with both conditions, and a higher level is frequently encountered in critically ill COVID-19 patients.

Fibrin split products (FSPs), which are one of the International Society of Thrombosis and Hemostasis (ISTH) criteria to diagnosis overt DIC, is often normal in milder COVID-19 illness. Levels of FSP can, however, be elevated in critically ill patients and have been associated with poor outcomes. Fibrinogen levels are often elevated in most patients with COVID-19 illness. In contrast, fibrinogen levels are low in patients with DIC. Similarly, PT and activated PTT (aPTT) is often normal in COVID-19 patients but is frequently elevated in DIC. Between PT and PTT, only PT prolongation is seen with the progression of COVID-19 illness.

Thrombocytopenia, which is another common finding in DIC and in critically ill septic patients, is uncommon in COVID-19 patients with only 5% of patients with platelet counts of <100 x 10^9/L. Thrombocytopenia, however, is common in patients with fatal COVID-19 and is seen in half of such cases. Nonetheless, progressive thrombocytopenia should prompt the workup for alternative etiologies such as bacterial superinfections and adverse drug reactions. (3)

Thromboelastogram (TEG) is another test designed to assess clot formation and dissolution. In a study evaluating incidence of a hypercoagulable state based on TEG and its association with thrombotic events noted that the hypercoagulable state was not associated with thrombotic events. Similarly, there was no association between hypercoagulable state and inflammatory markers, and coagulation markers and use of thromboprophylaxis. (4)

Like in any other illness, evaluation for a thrombotic state should start with a detailed history, physical examination, and results of laboratory tests for hemostasis. Patients with clinical suspicion for DVT should undergo further evaluation with venous Doppler or compression ultrasound examination. Similarly, PE should be considered if the patient is hypotensive or has unexplained hypoxia. Diagnosis relies on definitive imaging, as patients with COVID-19 can be hypoxic and present with signs of PE such as high D-dimers and right ventricular strain even in the absence of PE. Studies have shown that COVID-19 patients can have high incidence of thromboembolic events, especially when they have elevated hypercoagulability markers. Similarly, studies have shown the association between worsening coagulation markers and the development of cytokine storm and multiorgan failure.

Other macrovascular thrombotic conditions, such as myocardial injury or infarction, stroke, abdominal and thoracic aortic thrombosis, acute limb ischemia, and mesenteric ischemia, have also been reported in COVID-19 patients. Although stroke, aortic thrombosis, and acute limb ischemia can be diagnosed with a detailed physical examination and confirmed with diagnostic imaging, the diagnosis of other conditions can be particularly challenging in COVID-19 patients. For example, cardiac markers can be elevated in severe COVID-19 illness due to cytokine storm and hypoxic injury and not necessarily due to direct plaque rupture. Furthermore, typical chest pain is often absent in COVID-19 patients with acute coronary syndrome. Electrocardiogram (ECG) is often helpful as it can show ST elevation, whereas in those with equivocal symptoms and nonspecific EKG changes can benefit from echocardiogram and serial ECG monitoring. Mesenteric ischemia is uncommon, but it is another disease entity that can present with nonspecific findings such as abdominal pain, vomiting, or diarrhea. A routine CT with contrast could easily miss this diagnosis; especially early in the disease, and a dedicated CT angiography of mesenteric vessels is often needed for diagnosis. (5)

Treatment: Society guidelines have recommended prophylactic anticoagulation in all patients hospitalized with COVID-19 barring any contraindications. Mechanical prophylaxis has been recommended in patients with contraindications to chemical prophylaxis.

The American Society of Hematology (ASH) recommends using prophylactic-intensity over intermediate intensity or therapeutic-intensity anticoagulation in patients with COVID-19 without confirmed or suspected thromboembolic disease. Regarding specific anticoagulants for thromboprophylaxis, the American College of Chest Physicians (ACCP) guidelines recommend using standard dose LMWH or fondaparinux over unfractionated heparin (UFH) or direct oral anticoagulant therapy (DOAC; Table 3-1).

ASH and IISTH also favor LMWH therapy for thromboprophylaxis. Due to lack of data regarding benefits of extended prophylaxis after hospital discharge, ACCP has only recommended in-patient prophylaxis. For patients diagnosed with PE or proximal DVT, ACCP has favored LMWH over UFH to limit need for staff exposure and over DOAC due to their concern for drug interaction. ASH recommends either LMWH or UFH over DOAC therapy in these patients. ACCP also recommends a 20%-30% higher dose of LMWH for COVID-19 patients who develop recurrent VTE despite

TABLE 3-1 Anticoagulation Strategies in COVID-19 Patients

	Prevention	Treatment
Aspirin	No role to prevent VTE, may have role in preventing stroke and MI	First-line drug for stroke and MI, no role in VTE
Low molecular-weight-heparin	Preferred for VTE prophylaxis, less interactions, less staff exposure	Preferred for VTE treatment, less interactions, less staff exposure
Unfractionated heparin	May be used in ARDS patients (critically ill), not preferred	May be used in ARDS patients (critically ill), not preferred
DOACs	Can be used, but with caution due to drug-drug interaction	Can be used, but with caution due to drug-drug interaction
Parenteral thrombolytics	No role	Utilized for highly suspected/diagnosed cases with hemodynamic instability
Catheter-directed thrombolytics	No role	Utilized for highly suspected/diagnosed cases with hemodynamic instability

ARDS, acute respiratory disease syndrome; DOAC, direct oral anticoagulant; MI, myocardial infarct; VTE, venous thromboembolism.

appropriate weight-adjusted LMWH dosing. Antiplatelet therapy (e.g., aspirin) is likely inferior to anticoagulants for VTE prophylaxis in COVID-19 patients, but it has a definite role in the setting of stroke and MI.

Systemic thrombolysis is recommended by ACCP for VTE patients with hypotension (defined as systolic blood pressure of <90 mm Hg) or in those without hypotension who have progressive cardiopulmonary deterioration due to PE and have low risk for bleeding. (6)

In patients with acute limb ischemia, aortic thrombosis or mesenteric ischemia, a surgical or interventional radiology consultation is often required in addition to systemic anticoagulation. If there are signs of massive or high-risk PE with hemodynamic instability, a bedside echocardiogram followed by thrombolytic therapy is preferred. In case of refractory circulatory collapse or cardiac arrest, extracorporeal membrane oxygenation (ECMO) is an option of treatment, along with surgical embolectomy or catheter-directed treatment.

Management of stroke is similar to non-COVID patients with stroke, with IV alteplase therapy for patients without contraindications who are diagnosed within 3 hours of onset of symptoms or a select subgroup of patients presenting within 4.5 hours. Similarly, COVID-19 patients with ST elevation myocardial infarction (STEMI) are treated similar to non-COVID patients with STEMI. (1-5)

Prognosis and Monitoring: In a small series of patients with COVID infection receiving mechanical ventilation, systemic tPA (25 mg over 2 hours followed by another 25 mg over the subsequent 22 hours) was used. It showed improvement in ventilatory parameters, but the effect of this intervention on long-term outcomes is not known yet. (1-3) A second case series depicted the effect of aerosolized freeze-dried plasminogen in moderate to severe critically ill COVID-19 patients. The study reported great improvement in oxygenation and ventilatory parameters. (1-3) Although there have been many studies in this regard, the long-term role of thrombolytics is not clear.

ISTH and ASH are the only societies that recommend monitoring coagulation parameters such as D-dimer, PT, PTT, fibrinogen levels, and platelet count for risk stratification and for potential use of experimental therapies. ISTH recommends monitoring in all COVID-19 patients including those who are outpatients. ISTH also provides an algorithm based on these markers to assess which outpatients would benefit from inpatient therapy.

These markers include platelet count <100 x 10^9, fibrinogen level of <2.0 gm/L, three- to fourfold rise in D-dimer, and prolongation of PT. ISTH also recommends further evaluation of COVID-19 inpatients who have D-dimer levels of greater than six times above normal.

The Centers for Disease Control and Prevention (CDC) has stated that there is insufficient data to recommend for or against using these markers to guide management decisions. None of the societies have recommended daily use of these markers to guide anticoagulation dosing intensity. (6)

KEY POINTS

- Microvascular and macrovascular thrombosis is common in patients with COVID-19.
- In patients suspected to have thrombosis, evaluation should start with a detailed history, physical examination, and results of laboratory tests for hemostasis followed by confirmatory imaging.
- Treatment of thrombosis in COVID-19 is similar to non-COVID-19–associated thrombosis with the exception of the choice of anticoagulation agent. Most societies prefer using LMWH in COVID-19–associated thrombosis.

PATIENT EDUCATION

What is thrombosis?

Thrombosis of a body organ/part occurs when there is a blockage by the blood clot of one or more blood vessels that supply blood to that organ/part. For example, when a blockage occurs in blood vessels of the lung, it leads to thrombosis in the lung, also known as PE. Other types of thromboses that have been seen in COVID-19 illness include DVT (due to blockage of vein in the arms or legs), stroke (due to blockage of vessel in the brain), myocardial infarction (due to blockage of the vessels supplying the heart muscles), and mesenteric ischemia (due to blockage of the vessels supplying the gut).

What are the signs and symptoms?

When the blood clot blocks the blood vessels, it blocks the flow of blood through that organ or part of the body. If the blood clot blocks the lung (such as in PE) you can feel chest pain, dizziness, shortness of breath, or rapid heartbeat. If the blood clot blocks the vessels in the brain (such as in stroke), you can feel weakness or numbness of a part of the body. If the blood clot develops in leg veins, you can have pain, swelling, and redness in the involved leg. If the blood clot blocks the vessels in the heart (such as in myocardial infarction), you can feel chest pain that may radiate to your left arm and shortness of breath. If you develop any of these symptoms, immediately call 9-1-1.

How is it diagnosed and treated?

There are several tests that your provider can do to find out if you are have thrombosis in any part of your body. To find thrombosis in the lungs (PE) your provider may do a blood test, a CT of your chest, or a ventilation/perfusion scan (specialized test of your lungs to check if the blood supply is adequate in every part). Blood clot in the leg veins (DVT) can be diagnosed with the ultrasound of the legs, and blood clot in the brain (stroke) can be diagnosed with CT or magnetic resonance imaging (MRI) of the brain. Blood clot in the heart (myocardial infarction) can be diagnosed with a combination of ECG, blood test, and coronary angiogram (a test in which your doctor will insert a small tube into a large vein of your body and gently push it to your heart). The doctor will then inject a dye to check which vessel is blocked.

Blood clots are treated with anticoagulants (or blood thinners). You may receive a shot or a pill of blood thinner. These medications can increase the risk of bleeding, therefore please watch for any signs or symptoms such as dark stools, nasal or oral bleeding, coughing up blood, or feeling tired or dizzy (which can happen if you develop low blood counts due to bleeding). If you develop any of these signs, seek immediate medical attention. Your doctor may treat you with additional medications depending on the part of body where you develop clot, such as medications to lower your cholesterol, medications to block platelets (a blood cell that participates in clot formation), and medications to prevent change in size, mass, geometry, and function of heart after injury.

References

1. Wang X, Sahu KK, Cerny J. Coagulopathy, endothelial dysfunction, thrombotic microangiopathy and complement activation: potential role of complement system inhibition in COVID-19. *J Thromb Thrombolysis.* 2021;51(3):657-662.
2. Gasecka A, Borovac JA, Guerreiro RA, et al. Thrombotic complications in patients with COVID-19: pathophysiological mechanisms, diagnosis, and treatment. *Cardiovasc Drugs Ther.* 2021;35(2):215-229.
3. Hadid T, Kafri Z, Al-Katib A. Coagulation and anticoagulation in COVID-19. *Blood Rev.* 2020;Oct 8:100761.

4. Salem N, Atallah B, El Nekidy WS, Sadik ZG, Park WM, Mallat J. Thromboelastography findings in critically ill COVID-19 patients. *J Thromb Thrombolysis*. 2020;51(4):961-965.

5. Avila J, Long B, Holladay D, Gottlieb M. Thrombotic complications of COVID-19. *Am J Emerg Med*. 2021;39:213-218.

6. Flaczyk A, Rosovsky RP, Reed CT, et al. Comparison of published guidelines for management of coagulopathy and thrombosis in critically ill patients with COVID 19: implications for clinical practice and future investigations. *Crit Care*. 2020;24:559.

CHAPTER 4

COVID-19 and Heart Failure

MIGUEL RODRIGUEZ GUERRA,
MUHAMMAD K. GUHJJAR

CASE PRESENTATION

A 72-year-old Hispanic male with a history of hypertension was brought to the emergency department complaining of persistent fatigue and malaise and watery diarrhea associated with lightheadedness for 2 days. He has recently returned from Europe. He tried home remedies to control the diarrhea, but they did not help. No recent antibiotic use and he takes amlodipine for hypertension. Family history and social history were noncontributory. In the emergency department he was found to be febrile, otherwise, he had normal vitals. Physical examination was unremarkable. Laboratory data showed prerenal azotemia, elevated lactate dehydrogenase (LDH), and low leukocyte count. He was transferred to the medical floor for intravenous hydration and further workup. On the floor, SARS-CoV-2 polymerase chain reaction was confirmed. The next day he suddenly became hypotensive and developed severe respiratory distress. Chest radiograph (CXR) showed acute pulmonary edema. He was moved to critical care and started on noninvasive ventilation. His pro-brain natriuretic peptide (BNP) and troponin were elevated, and his renal function further worsened. Transthoracic echocardiogram (TTE) showed moderately reduced left ventricular (LV) function with global wall motion abnormalities. No prior echocardiogram was available. He was later mechanically ventilated and started on pressors. The patient underwent right heart catheterization that showed low cardiac output and elevated pulmonary capillary wedge pressure indicating cardiogenic shock. He continued to require inotropes and vasopressors. The patient also received tocilizumab and remdesivir for a total of 5 days, broad-spectrum antibiotics for a total of 7 days, as well as supportive measures. After 5 days of mechanical ventilation, the patient started to show improvement and was weaned off from the ventilator and renal function started to improve. After 12 days of hospitalization the patient was discharged home on carvedilol 6.25 mg and lisinopril 5 mg. Two months post-discharge, he presented to the cardiology clinic for a follow-up; repeat echocardiogram showed improved LV function.

Epidemiology: COVID-19 has been associated with various cardiovascular complications that may include subclinical myocardial injury, de novo heart failure (HF), and worsening of existing HF. Several observational studies from China, Europe, and the United States have reported the prevalence of HF in COVID-19 patients ranging from 4%-12%.[1] HF in COVID-19 patients has been associated with exceedingly high mortality. Older age group and people with preexisting HF has a higher chance of complications with this infection. In a recent global observational study, coronary artery disease (CAD) and congestive heart failure (CHF) are considered the predictors of inpatient mortality. Although the data on difference in outcomes in heart failure with reduced ejection fraction (HFrEF) and heart failure with preserved ejection fraction (HFpEF) are limited, clinical progression of disease remains similar in both cohorts. (1-3)

Pathophysiology: COVID-19 infection can lead to acute inflammatory response like other viral infections and may lead to decompensated HF. The cytokine storm can cause further worsening of cardiac function by demand-supply mismatch that ultimately manifests as HF exacerbation. Another important aspect is the malfunction of coagulation cascade that leads to prothrombotic effects, causing further myocardial damage at a macrovascular/microvascular level. COVID-19 may lead to direct myocardial injury that presents as fulminant myocarditis causing cardiogenic shock. The renin-angiotensin-aldosterone system (RAAS) system activation as a cause and effect of viral infection flares up the worsening of already affected myocardium.

TABLE 4-1 Causes of Heart Failure Exacerbation Due to COVID-19

Inflammatory response	New onset and worsening of heart failure
Coagulopathy	Microvascular dysfunction/cardiomyopathy/RV failure
RAAS activation	LV remodeling, fluid overload state
Sympathetic stimulation	Stress-induced cardiomyopathy
Lung parenchymal disease	Pulmonary hypertension
Direct cardiac injury	Acute myocarditis

LV, left ventricle; RAAS, renin-angiotensin-aldosterone system; RV, right ventricle.

Another manifestation of sepsis related to viral infection is sympathetic pathway activation leading to stress-induced cardiomyopathy. Right ventricular (RV) failure due to either thromboembolic disorder or direct viral infection can further worsen the disease process (Table 4-1).

PRESENTATION

The symptomatology of COVID-19 pneumonia and HF are overlapping, and all HF patients should be screened for COVIID infection. Fever, hypoxemia, cough, dyspnea, anosmia, tachycardia, and pulmonary rales and crackles are the initial signs/symptoms. The presence of nasal congestion, muscle aches, and diarrhea hints more toward COVID-19 infection. Similarly, the presence of jugular venous distention (JVD), S3, and exertional dyspnea are hallmark findings in HF.

DIAGNOSTIC MODALITIES

Electrocardiogram (ECG) is the initial diagnostic test which varies from sinus tachycardia to any arrhythmia, such as bigeminy, and nonsustained ventricular tachycardia to atrial fibrillation. Prolonged QTc is a common ECG finding in HF patients with COVID-19 infection. CXR may show pulmonary edema and enlarged cardiac silhouette. Chest computed tomography (CT) may show interstitial edema, ground-glass opacities, and pleural effusion.

Cardiac biomarkers such as troponin and pro-BNP elevation point toward myocardial injury and have a prognostic role in HF patients. They may be elevated in the setting of acute respiratory distress syndrome (ARDS), acute kidney injury, and thromboembolic disease. Inflammatory markers such as C-reactive protein (CRP), ferritin, and interleukin (IL)-6 are elevated in COVID-19 infection and are considered markers of a worse prognosis. In observational studies, persistent elevation of D-dimer, IL-6, troponin, and LDH has been linked to remarkably high mortality. Markers of inflammation and thrombogenicity are measured every 2-3 days to risk stratify patients.

TTE is an essential tool to assess cardiac functions in COVID-19-related HF and its complications. Myocardial edema, LV dysfunction, worsening of valvular disease, RV dysfunction, pulmonary hypertension, and decreased global longitudinal strain are pertinent echocardiographic findings. Coronary angiography/CT angiography and magnetic resonance imaging (MRI) are considered if myocarditis is suspected based on availability to diagnose and risk stratify the disease.

THERAPEUTICS AND COMPLICATIONS

Management of HF in COVID-19 infection is a complex process. The algorithm starts from better fluid status assessment and monitoring vital signs. This can be performed noninvasively either by careful clinical exam, inferior vena cava (IVC) diameter/collapsibility measurement, and E/e' assessment or invasively by hemodynamic assessment by pulmonary artery catheter. Patients with HF and COVID-19 are at higher risk of hypotension, which is why judicious use of diuretics and fluids should be guided by objective findings.

Diuretics: Use of diuretics to achieve euvolemia is key, but the dose should be adjusted to avoid dehydration. Concomitant sepsis and gastrointestinal (GI) bleeding should be considered to avoid hypoperfusion. Use of nonsteroidal anti-inflammatory drugs (NSAIDs) should be avoided to prevent kidney injury in combination with diuretics.

ACE-I/ARBS/ARNI: SARS-CoV-2 invades the lung cells by binding to angiotensin-converting enzyme 2 (ACE2) and can affect angiotensin levels in the tissue. It has been hypothesized that the use of angiotensin-converting enzyme inhibition (ACE-I) can interfere with the angiotensin levels, upregulating ACE2 and worsening COVID-19 infection in patients on ACE-I/angiotensin receptive blockers (ARBs). Several observational studies have indicated that ACE-I/ARBs have no role in the worsening of COVID-19 disease and may be protective at later stages of the disease. Thus, ACE-I/ARB/angiotensin receptor-neprilysin inhibitor (ARNI) should not be withheld in patients with COVID-19 infection and efforts to avoid hypotension should be made. In fact, the dose can be reduced if persistent hypotension is expected to avoid renal complications.

Beta Blocker: Although beta blockers have been considered as a standard-of-care treatment in HF, care should be taken in patients with COVID-19 infection. Because fever and tachycardia are commonly observed in these patients, special attention should be paid to avoid suppression of physiologic response and the dose of beta blocker should be adjusted based on hemodynamic assessment. Another aspect of treatment is the use of antiviral agents, such as darunavir. These agents may cause hypotension and bradycardia, so the dose of beta blockers can be reduced. Carvedilol has been hypothesized to have an anti-cytokine role, which needs to be validated.

MRA: Although the data regarding continuation of mineralocorticoid receptor antagonist (MRA) in HF patients with COVID-19 infection is limited, the general consensus is to avoid its use in the setting of renal complications and electrolyte abnormalities.

COVID-19-Specific Drugs and HF Medications: Use of antiviral medications, azithromycin, and hydroxychloroquine should be monitored, especially in view of drug-drug interactions. Prolonged QTc can lead to sudden cardiac death. Care should be taken specifically when patients are using antiarrhythmic and anticoagulation medications to avoid complications.

Respiratory Management: Patients with HF and COVID-19 infection are at higher risk of hypoxia due to lung injury and pulmonary edema. Use of noninvasive ventilation and prone positioning can be utilized to alleviate the work of breathing in pulmonary edema, but care should be taken in concomitant ARDS to avoid further lung injury. Hence, early intubation and mechanical ventilation should be carried out promptly with lung-protective strategies.

Vasoactive/Inotropic Medications: Use of inotropes and vaso-pressors should be guided by appropriate hemodynamic assessment. There are no data regarding the use of inodilators in the setting of COVID-19 infection; hence, they can be used on case-by-case basis.

Mechanical Circulatory Support Devices: Veno-venous-extracorporeal membrane oxygenation (V-V ECMO) can be utilized in the setting of persistent hypoxemia despite mechanical ventilation. Intra-aortic balloon pump (IABP) and an Impella heart pump can be utilized in the setting of cardiogenic shock.

Management of HFpEF. Limited data have shown that patients with COVID-19 infection are at high risk for development of HFpEF in the long term.[2] This is due to the inflammation-related cardiac fibrosis that may lead to diastolic dysfunction and pulmonary hypertension. Management strategies remain similar, but care should be sought to control hypertension and other risk factors to prevent disease pro-gression (Figure 4-1).

PROGNOSIS AND MONITORING

Although COVID-19 in HF patients has been linked to adverse outcomes, understanding the disease process with careful monitor-ing is the cornerstone of long-term outcomes. These patients are at risk of development of HFpEF and cardiomyopathy. The long-term outcome of myocarditis is unknown and may vary from complete reversibility of LV function to irreversible damage.

Home monitoring in HF patients is difficult with virtual office visits because of the necessary assessment of fluid status. Therefore, care should be given to vital signs, intake/output charting, and patient education. Pulmonary artery monitoring system can be uti-lized in cases with complex hemodynamics (Figure 4-2).

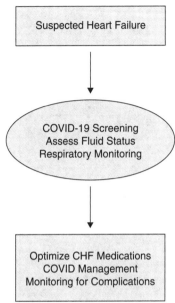

FIGURE 4-1 **Management algorithm of heart failure and COVID.**

KEY POINTS

- COVID-19 has been associated with various cardiovascular complications, which may include subclinical myocardial injury, de novo HF, and worsening of existing HF.
- Management of HF in COVID-19 infection is a complex process. The algorithm starts from better fluid status assessment and monitoring of vital signs.
- Pulmonary artery monitoring can be utilized in cases with complex hemodynamics.

PATIENT EDUCATION

Does HF put me at risk of COVID-19 infection?

HF patients are among the vulnerable groups who may have diseases that lead to worsening COVID-19 infection. Prevention is

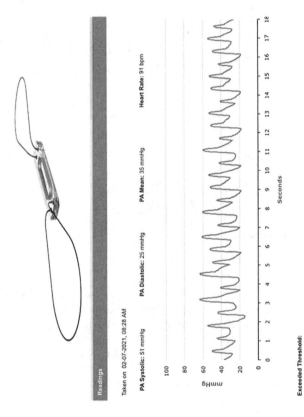

Readings

Taken on 02-07-2021, 08:28 AM

PA Systolic: 51 mmHg   PA Diastolic: 25 mmHg   PA Mean: 35 mmHg   Heart Rate: 91 bpm

Exceeded Threshold:

- Exceeded the PA Systolic Pressure threshold by 16
- Exceeded the PA Diastolic Pressure threshold by 5
- Exceeded the PA Mean Pressure threshold by 10
- Exceeded the Heart Rate threshold by 1

This reading was
marked approved by
the system

FIGURE 4-2 **CardioMEMS device for remote pulmonary artery (PA) pressure measurement in HF patients.**

the key, and care should be taken to avoid unnecessary social gatherings. A mask should be worn at all times. Symptoms such as cough, shortness of breath, nocturnal awakening with shortness of breath, and leg swelling should be reported to the physician.

How can I manage HF if I cannot go to see my doctor?

COVID-19 infection has been associated with worse outcomes in HF patients; hence, care should be taken to prevent infection. Medication and dietary compliance is the cornerstone of management. Daily weight and intake/output should be closely monitored. Telehealth visits can be performed if there is any concern regarding medications and symptoms.

References

1. Bader F, Manla Y, Atallah B, Starling RC. Heart failure and COVID-19. *Heart Fail Rev.* 2021;26:1-10.
2. Freaney PM, Shah SJ. COVID-19 and heart failure with preserved ejection fraction. *JAMA.* 2020. [Online ahead of print.] doi: 10.1001/jama.2020.17445.
3. Zhang Y, Coats AJS, Zheng Z,et al. Management of heart failure patients with COVID-19: a joint position paper of the Chinese Heart Failure Association & National Heart Failure Committee and the Heart Failure Association of the European Society of Cardiology. *Eur J Heart Fail.* 2020;22(6):941-956.

CHAPTER 5

COVID-19 and Cardiac Arrhythmias

JEIRYM MIRANDA TEJADA,
TIMOTHY J. VITTORIO

CASE PRESENTATION

A 59-year-old male presented to the emergency department with complaints of fever, cough, and progressive shortness of breath for the last 8 days. Initially, it began as flu-like symptoms with cephalgia, myalgia, and dry cough. Despite over-the-counter usage of acetaminophen and cough syrup, the symptoms worsened. Due to anorexia, he lost 8 lb. Additionally, he noticed pain and swelling in the right lower extremity. He works as a corporate counselor and has frequently traveled to Europe for business meetings and mentions his wife had similar symptoms, which improved after 1 week. The past medical history includes hypertension and hyperlipidemia, treated with lisinopril and atorvastatin, respectively. He denied any toxic habits. There was no past surgical history. On physical examination, he was noted to be in acute distress; tachypneic; and with dry, pale mucous membranes. The vital signs showed a blood pressure of 157/89 mmHg, heart rate 115 beats/min, respiratory rate 26 breaths/min, temperature 103.1°F, and SpO_2 89% with an air flow rate of 4 L/min. Bilateral dry rales were noted diffusely over the lung fields. Tachycardia was present. There was a normal S1, increased P2, and grade II/VI holosystolic murmur at the lower left parasternal border. The right lower extremity was warm, tender, and edematous. The remaining physical examination was unremarkable (Table 5-1).

The 12-lead electrocardiograms (ECGs) are shown in Figure 5-1A and B.

TABLE 5-1 Laboratory Values

WBC: 15.5 k/μL	BUN: 22 mg/dL
Neutrophils: 80.7%	Creatinine: 1.0 mg/dL
Lymphocytes: 16.1%	Calcium: 6.7 mg/dL
Hemoglobin: 15 g/dL	AST: 31 unit/L
Hematocrit: 45.4%	ALT: 37 unit/L
Platelets: 121 k/μL	Total bilirubin: 0.5 mg/dL
D-dimer: 1505 ng/mL	Direct bilirubin: 0.2 mg/dL
Sodium: 153 mEq/L	LDH: 713 unit/L
Potassium: 2.3 mEq/L	CRP: 98 mg/L
Glucose: 222 mg/dL	Pro-BNP: 3576 pg/mL
Chloride 109 mEq/L	Troponin: 84 ng/L
Bicarbonate: 29 mEq/L	Lactic acid: 5.6 mmoles/L

Sinus tachycardia, left axis deviation, short PR interval, and ST-T wave changes in the precordial leads are suggestive of anterior wall ischemia and prolonged QTc interval.

Chest computed tomography (CT) Scan: Small bilateral effusions with near complete collapse of the right lower lobe. Nonspecific ground-glass opacity in the lingula may represent atypical pneumonia (Figure 5-2).

Transthoracic echocardiogram (TTE) showed normal left ventricle size and systolic function. There was moderate tricuspid regurgitation with moderately elevated pulmonary artery systolic pressure.

A venous Doppler duplex ultrasound of the bilateral lower extremities revealed acute deep vein thrombosis of the right superficial femoral vein.

He was placed on high-flow oxygen therapy and treated with intravenous azithromycin, cefepime, and vancomycin. The patient received hydroxychloroquine (HCQ) and low-molecular–weight heparin for anticoagulation. The electrolyte and metabolic derangements were corrected.

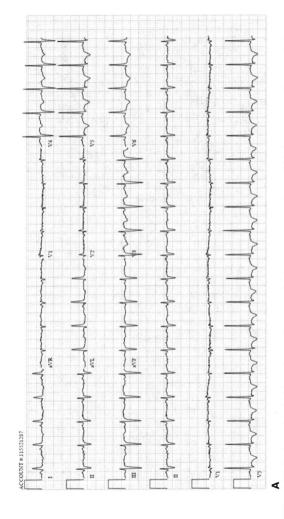

ACCOUNT #115531287

A

FIGURE 5-1 **(A) (B).** Sinus tachycardia, left axis deviation, short PR interval, and ST-T wave changes in the precordial leads are suggestive of anterior wall ischemia and prolonged QTc interval.

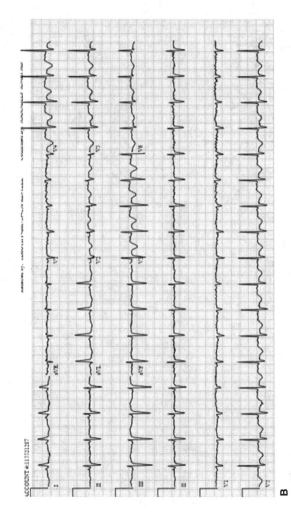

FIGURE 5-1 (*Continued*)

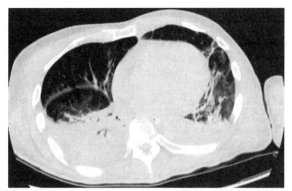

FIGURE 5-2 **CT scan chest showing bilateral imfiltrates with pleural effusion.**

A nasopharyngeal swab was performed and SARS-CoV-2 was detected by real-time reverse-transcriptase polymerase chain reaction (rRT-PCR).

After 3 weeks of hospitalization, the patient clinically improved and was discharged to a short-term rehabilitation facility.

INTRODUCTION

A major global health concern has emerged from the rapid spreading of coronavirus disease 2019 (COVID-19), which is caused by the severe acute respiratory syndrome coronavirus 2 (SARS-CoV-2). It was first reported in Wuhan, Hubei Province, China, on December 2019. Millions of cases have been reported worldwide, impacting global health and economy. Although it primarily affects the respiratory tract, other organs are concurrently involved such as the cardiovascular system, significantly affecting cardiac function and conduction system, which is associated with increased disease severity and adverse outcomes. As new data emerge, our knowledge about the impact of COVID-19 on cardiac arrhythmias continues to evolve and further studies are required for better understanding of its pathophysiology and management strategies.

Epidemiology: One aspect of cardiac injury among COVID-19 patients and overall critical illness is an increased risk for cardiac arrhythmias. These were first described by Wang and colleagues, reporting a 17% (23/138) incidence of arrhythmias; 16 patients were admitted to the intensive care unit (ICU), accounting for 44% of the total number of ICU patients. A recent study revealed normal 12-lead ECGs on only 26% of the patients. Lei and associates reported 24% of arrhythmias in COVID-19 patients, and 33% of ICU admitted patients had developed arrhythmias. (1) In fatal cases of COVID-19, 60% developed arrhythmias, and additionally, cardiac arrhythmias were independently associated with an increased risk of in-hospital mortality (11.5% vs. 5.6% among those patients without arrhythmia; odds ratio, 1.95; 95% confidence interval [CI], 1.33-2.86). In clinically stable patients, a low prevalence of arrhythmias was noted.

In the United States, the data on arrhythmia characterization in COVID-19 patients are now emerging. Recent published cases from New York observed several manifestations of arrhythmias varying from bradyarrhythmias including transient complete heart block (CHB) and high-degree atrioventricular (AV) block, to tachyarrhythmias including supraventricular tachycardia (SVT) and atrial fibrillation/flutter (AF/flutter), as well as ventricular arrhythmias such as monomorphic or polymorphic ventricular tachycardia (VT) and sudden cardiac arrest (SCA) with pulseless electrical activity (PEA).

QTc prolongation leading to torsades de pointes (TdP) was commonly reported in association with various conditions such as electrolyte and metabolic derangements, certain drugs used in the treatment of COVID-19 disease, myocarditis toxicity, and inherited arrhythmia syndromes. Furthermore, a case of Brugada-type pattern 12-lead ECG was present that later resulted in a brief episode of AV nodal reentrant tachycardia (AVNRT).

These manifestations suggest various potential mechanisms for arrhythmogenesis.

Pathophysiology: The specific cause of arrhythmias among COVID-19 patients has not been specified, but potential mechanisms include not only the direct viral effect but also systemic illness including hypoxia, abnormal host immunologic response, myocarditis, myocardial strain, myocardial ischemia, drug interactions and side effects, electrolyte disorders, and intravascular volume imbalance.

The effects of these mechanisms can cause an exacerbation of a previous underlying cardiomyopathy and conduction disorder or induce new electrophysiological abnormalities in patients without any previous history of cardiac disease.

Hypoxia. Lung injury from COVID-19 leads to acute respiratory failure and hypoxemia, which is known to cause hypoxia-induced cellular damage activating anaerobic glycolysis, reducing intracellular pH, and increasing intracellular calcium levels and extracellular levels facilitating early and late depolarization and alterations in the action potential (AP) duration.

Abnormal host immune response. Several cytokines including interleukin (IL)-6, tumor necrosis factor (TNF)-α, and IL-1 can modulate the expression and function of calcium and potassium channels (inflammatory cardiac channelopathies) causing prolongation of ventricular APs, along with direct myocardial injury. These cytokines cause overactivation of the cardiac sympathetic system using the hypothalamus-mediated inflammatory reflex and peripheral-mediated activation of the stellate ganglion pathway, which can lead to QTc interval prolongation. Cytokines are well known arrhythmogenic triggers, especially in patients with underlying long QT syndrome (LQTS). Furthermore, IL-6 increases the bioavailability of QTc interval–prolonging drugs by inhibition of cytochrome P450 (CYP450).

Myocarditis. The pathophysiology of myocarditis can be explained by a possible mechanism that includes direct myocardial injury due to direct viral tissue involvement or due to extrapulmonary migration of infected alveolar macrophages. It can potentially predispose a patient to enhanced arrhythmogenic risk by disrupting electrical conduction. SARS-CoV-2 binds to angiotensin-converting enzyme 2 (ACE2) receptors on the myocardial cell membrane by utilizing the spike protein. In theory, when SARS-CoV-2 attaches to the ACE2 receptors found on the myocardium, there is downregulation of ACE2 receptors, causing unopposed angiotensin II accumulation, which leads to adverse myocardial remodeling by its action on angiotensin II type 1 receptors.

Another possible mechanism is via cell-mediated cytotoxicity in which primed $CD8^+$ T lymphocytes migrate to the cardiomyocytes and cause myocardial inflammation. Via cytokine storm or cytokine release syndrome, proinflammatory cytokines are released into the circulation, augmenting T-lymphocyte activation that further releases more cytokines and results in a positive feedback loop of immune activation and myocardial injury.

Myocarditis may cause arrhythmia in the acute stage as a consequence of the direct cytopathic effect, producing electrical imbalances, ischemia from microvascular dysfunction, and dysfunction of gap junctions from impaired myocardial expression of connexins. It also may cause ion-channel impairment, which is especially seen in patients with overlapping inflammatory channelopathies.

In viral myocarditis, factors from the host and virus can cause structural as well as electrophysiological remodeling, causing abnormal calcium handling and downregulation of potassium channels, leading to prolonged repolarization and abnormal conduction. Prolonged repolarization can induce triggered activity, whereas in combination with abnormal conduction (which involves reduced conduction velocity, decreased refractoriness, and increased diffusion of conduction in the myocardium) can cause either circus-type reentry or phase 2 reentry without an obstacle. Arrhythmias can also be seen in the postinflammatory stage, promoted by the presence of variable degrees of myocardial scarring.

Myocardial ischemia. Myocardial injury with ST-segment elevation has been reported in patients with COVID-19 infection. Microvascular dysfunction and hyperinflammatory state are potential causes for myocardial ischemia by leading to activation of inflammatory cells and a cytokine surge within a preexisting atherosclerotic plaque. This causes vasoconstriction due to dysregulation of the coronary vascular endothelium, which can result in acute coronary syndrome (ACS). IL-6 and TNF-α can both cause depletion of the coagulation and fibrinolytic system, leading to bleeding as well as thrombosis, and promote microvascular dysfunction in the form of disseminated intravascular coagulation (DIC). Another possible mechanism of microvascular dysfunction causing myocardial ischemia is infection-mediated vasculitis triggered as a result of a hypersensitivity reaction induced by direct viral entry in the myocardial endothelial cells or due to indirect immunological response.

Myocardial strain. The most common reported thrombotic complication in COVID-19 patients is pulmonary embolism and, along with pulmonary hypertension, causes severe acute respiratory distress syndrome (ARDS), heart failure (HF), or sepsis. They can result in an increase of right-sided cardiac filling pressures leading to right myocardial strain. In these patients, there is an increased risk of atrial tachyarrhythmias as a result of increased right atrial pressure and an increased sympathetic tone. A case was reported in a patient who was found to have a temporary occurrence of S1Q3T3 12-lead ECG pattern who later developed transient CHB suggested to be caused by pulmonary arterial hypertension.

Drug side effects. Several antimicrobial drugs that are currently being used as potential "off-label" therapeutic agents for COVID-19 have uncertain benefits, yet they are either known to induce or may induce QTc interval prolongation with potential ventricular proarrhythmic effects such as TdP. These agents are chloroquine (CQ), HCQ, azithromycin, and lopinavir/ritonavir. Recent evidence indicates significant QTc interval prolongation in COVID-19 patients receiving HCQ alone or concomitantly with azithromycin. Advanced AV conduction block was also observed. HCQ and azithromycin inhibit the hERG-K^+ channel causing prolongation of the AP, and with unopposed inward Na^+ and Ca^{2+} currents they trigger early after depolarization (EAD) leading to TdP. The cardiac effects with other therapies used in COVID-19 including ribavirin, remdesivir, and tocilizumab remain uncertain because there are no sufficient data.

Electrolyte derangements. It has been well studied that the effect of electrolyte abnormalities including hypokalemia, hypomagnesemia, and hypophosphatemia is a precipitant for preexistent or new-onset arrhythmias. Electrolyte disturbances were observed in 7.2% of 416 hospitalized patients with COVID-19 infection reported in a case series, and they were attributed to COVID-19–associated acute renal injury or diarrhea.

Intravascular volume imbalance. Intravascular volume imbalance is commonly encountered in critically ill patients as well as in COVID-19 due to either sepsis caused from ARDS, HF, or a combination of both. AF appears to be the most commonly encountered arrhythmia in the critical care setting.

Diagnostic: The majority of patients present with a systemic illness consistent with COVID-19, rather than specific signs or symptoms of arrhythmias or conduction system disease. The patients may be tachycardic (with or without palpitation) in the setting of other illness-related symptoms (e.g., fever, pain, shortness of breath, etc.)

Physicians should be cognizant of potential rhythm disturbances in COVID-19 patients. Therefore, it is necessary to have a baseline examination and to determine essential clinical information, such as a history of palpitation, dizziness, arrhythmias, unexplained syncope, family history of premature sudden cardiac death (SCD), and a detailed medication history, especially medications that might cause 12-lead ECG QTc interval prolongation, to evaluate those patients who may be at higher risk for cardiac arrhythmias.

Cardiovascular Testing:
12-lead ECG. A baseline 12-lead ECG showed be performed at the time of admission on most patients suspected of COVID-19. Although nonessential testing, including serial ECGs, should be avoided to reduce exposure of front-line medical workers and other patients to infectious risk, the ECG should be closely monitored for early warning, intervention and especially in patients with cardiac comorbidities and in whom QTc interval prolonging medications are planned to be used. Physicians should identify any ST-T wave changes accompanied by continuous dynamic changes in two or more leads with R wave domination, abnormal Q waves, continuous, coupled, polymorphic or multifocal premature ventricular contractions (PVCs); new-onset sinus, AV conduction block, complete left or right bundle branch block (LBBB or RBBB), sinus arrest; AF/ flutter, AVNRT and low-voltage or wide QRS complexes.

Continuous ECG monitoring and transthoracic echocardiography. These modalities are not required for all patients unless there is a development of cardiac manifestations, documented cardiac arrhythmias, suspected myocardial ischemia or other standard indications.

Therapeutics: The management of any bradyarrhythmia or tachyarrhythmia in the setting of COVID-19 infection is no different from the routine management of these conditions without COVID-19 infection and should include optimization of supportive treatments, identifying and correcting secondary causes such as electrolyte or metabolic imbalances, myocardial ischemia, hypoxia, fever and pro-arrhythmic effects of drugs. The goal is to safely treat by limiting exposure and focusing on the transient nature of arrhythmias and drug-drug interactions (Table 5-2).

Bradyarrhythmias. Isoprenaline and atropine can be used in patients with persistent bradycardia and should be considered prior to the implantation of a temporary transvenous pacemaker. Given the transient nature of bradyarrhythmias, nature of critical illness, risk of bacterial superinfection, and risk of device infection, prior to implanting a permanent device, temporary pacemaker implantation is considered reasonable. The evaluation of a permanent pacemaker should be reassessed after recovery from COVID-19 infection.

Atrial tachyarrhythmias. For acute termination in patients with SVT, intravenous adenosine can be used and synchronized electrical cardioversion can be considered in patients with refractory cases; it should be postponed in asymptomatic and stable patients. Maintenance therapy with β-adrenoceptor (BBs) or calcium-channel antagonists (CCBs) may be initiated if there are no contraindications. Drug-drug interactions with antiviral agents must be evaluated prior to initiation of these medications to avoid the risk of bradycardia and QTc interval prolongation.

Similarly, patients with new-onset of AF/flutter with a stable rhythm can be treated with rate control. Rhythm-control strategy should be reserved for patients with hemodynamically unstable patients or in HF patients. It can be achieved with synchronized electrical cardioversion or antiarrhythmic drugs (AADs) such as amiodarone. There is a high risk of immediate arrhythmia recurrence without the use of any AAD as maintenance therapy, which

TABLE 5-2 COVID and Cardiac Arrhythmias

Arrhythmias	• Bradyarrhythmia
	• Supraventricular tachycardia
	• Atrial fibrillation
	• Atrial flutter
	• Heart blocks
	• Ventricular tachyarrhythmias
	• Sudden cardiac arrest
Mechanism	• Hypoxia
	• Drug interactions and side effects
	• Myocardial ischemia
	• Myocarditis
	• Myocardial strain
	• Electrolytes disarrangement
	• Abnormal host immune response
Diagnostic	• Clinical history and physical examination
	• 12-lead ECG
	• ±Continuous cardiac monitoring
	• ±Transthoracic echocardiogram
Management	Generalized management like non–COVID-19 patients.
	• Identify and treat secondary causes (electrolyte or metabolic imbalances, myocardial ischemia, hypoxia, fever, and proarrhythmic effects of drugs).
	• Monitor baseline ECG, QTc interval, K^+, Mg^{2+}, Ca^{2+}, and PO_4^{2-}.
	• Bradyarrhythmia: atropine, isoprenaline, temporary pacemaker. Need for permanent pacemaker should be reassessed after recovery.
	• Atrial tachyarrhythmias: rate control or rhythm control.
	• Ventricular arrhythmias: antiarrhythmic drugs and/or electrical defibrillation.
	• Special management for patient with inherited conduction disorders.
	• Minimize healthcare and patient exposure.
	• Triaging EP procedures.

ECG, electrocardiogram; EP, electrophysiology.

can be minimized by treating secondary causes of arrhythmias prior to attempting rhythm-control strategy. Once hemodynamically stable, discontinuation of AADs should be considered given serious drug-drug interactions with antiviral drugs and rate-controlling medications started with BBs or CCBs unless contraindicated, with or without digoxin. In terms of anticoagulation, there are data suggesting that COVID-19 infection might be associated with a hypercoagulable state, increasing the risk for thromboembolism. After recovering from COVID-19 infection, a rate- versus rhythm-control strategy should be reassessed along with the need for anticoagulation.

Ventricular arrhythmias. If the patient develops sustained VT, intravenous infusion of amiodarone and other antiarrhythmic medications may be administered, but external defibrillation can be used if necessary. If ventricular fibrillation (VF) occurs, then advanced cardiac life support (ACLS) protocol must be implemented with immediate defibrillation.

Arrhythmia-related procedures. The Heart Rhythm Society COVID-19 Task Force has created a consensus document that divides electrophysiological procedures into urgent or emergent, semi-urgent, and nonurgent or elective procedures. Emergent procedures are considered if they reduce the risk of clinical deterioration, hospitalization, or death. Elective and nonurgent procedures should be postponed until a later date to minimize the potential exposure of healthcare personnel. Conversely, urgent and semi-urgent procedures should be performed if the perceived benefits of the procedure to the patient outweigh the risks of resource utilization and healthcare personnel exposure. (1-5)

Monitoring/follow-up. It is recommended to obtain a pretreatment baseline 12-lead ECG, QTc interval measurement, and baseline electrolytes (K^+, Ca^{2+}, and Mg^{2+}) to determine high-risk cardiovascular and comorbid conditions.

A dynamic discussion with the patient about the benefits and risks of receiving any QTc interval–prolonging medications should be ongoing based on the baseline risk perceived or actual benefit of therapy and development of significant QTc interval prolongation or TdP.

Reevaluation of the risk of TdP, discontinuation of other QTc interval–prolonging medications, and correction of all electrolyte abnormalities is recommended, as well as placing the patient on continuous telemetry or mobile 12-lead ECG devices, with consideration of a wearable defibrillator (LifeVest) or placement of external defibrillator patches.

After recovery from COVID-19 infection, evaluation of a permanent pacemaker and automatic implantable cardioverter defibrillator therapies should be reassessed.

KEY POINTS

- Pay attention to any cardiac arrhythmias in COVID-19 patients that might be more common in critically ill patients.
- Arrhythmias are thought to be a result of not only the direct viral effect but also due to systemic illness, drug interactions, and side effects. SARS-CoV-2 may induce electrophysiological abnormalities in patients without a previous history of heart disease or cause exacerbation of underlying cardiomyopathy and conduction disorders.
- Arrhythmia should be regarded as one of the main complications of COVID-19, and early diagnosis, proactive monitoring, and timely treatment to reduce mortality is crucial.
- Optimizing supportive management strategies and minimizing exposure to COVID-19 infection are imperative.
- More data and studies are required to better understand the pathophysiology and to validate management strategies.

PATIENT EDUCATION

What are the symptoms of arrhythmias in COVID-19?
People can have dizziness, sensation of fast heart beats, loss of consciousness, chest pain, and nonspecific symptoms like fever, cough, and trouble breathing.

How can it be diagnosed?

You should see a doctor if you present with any of the symptoms mentioned above or have a history of a heart condition. Your doctor can order a 12-lead ECG and heart monitor.

How can the arrhythmias be treated?

It is very important to control the fever, provide oxygen therapy, and maintain adequate hydration and electrolytes, such as potassium, calcium, magnesium, and phosphorus, within normal levels. Medications that can cause or worsen abnormal heart rhythms should be discontinued, avoided, or changed to an alternative.

References

1. Lei S, Jiang F, Su W, et al. Clinical characteristics and outcomes of patients undergoing surgeries during the incubation period of COVID-19 infection. *EClinicalMedicine*. 2020;21:100331.
2. Dherange P, Lang J, Qian P, et al. Arrhythmias and COVID-19: a review. *J Am Coll Cardiol EP*. 2020;6(9):1193-1204.
3. Prutkin JM. COVID-19: arrhythmias and conduction system disease. *UpToDate*. 2021.
4. Kochav SM, Coromilas E, Nalbandian A, et al. Cardiac arrhythmias in COVID-19 infection. *Circ Arrhythm Electrophysiol*. 2020;13:3008719.
5. Yueying Wang MS, Zhaojia Wang MS, Tse G, et al. Cardiac arrhythmias in patients with COVID-19. *J Arrhythm*. 2020;36(5):827-836.

CHAPTER 6

COVID-19 and Valvular Heart Disease

RISHI SHRIVASTAV, AMANDEEP SINGH

CASE PRESENTATION

A 78-year-old female patient with history of type 2 diabetes mellitus, hypertension, and moderate aortic stenosis (AS) on a transthoracic echocardiogram (TTE) done 1 year ago is brought to a New York City hospital with fever, fatigue, cough, and worsening dyspnea in April 2020. On arrival the patient was found to be tachypneic, hypoxic, and tachycardic. Physical examination showed an elderly female responding to verbal stimuli but in distress with increased work of breathing. Respiratory exam revealed intercostal retractions and diffusely coarse breath sounds along with crackles in both lung fields. Auscultatory findings consisted of tachycardia, with a late peaking systolic murmur that would radiate to bilateral carotid arteries. Abdomen was soft and nontender, but extremities revealed 1+ pitting edema with cold extremities. The decision was made to intubate the patient and start her on mechanical ventilation. Investigation pursued thereafter showed leukocytosis of 21,000 with predominant neutrophilia and lymphopenia. Metabolic panel revealed elevated blood, urea, nitrogen (BUN) and creatinine to 40 and 2.0, respectively, with unknown prior baseline. The CO_2 was at 18, but the electrolytes were normal. A portable chest X-ray showed diffuse bilateral interstitial opacities with small bilateral pleural effusions concerning for bilateral pneumonia and congestive heart failure. Electrocardiogram (ECG) showed sinus tachycardia with voltage criteria of left ventricular hypertrophy. Patient was transferred to the intensive care unit (ICU) where she was put in airborne precautions for concerns of COVID-19 disease. Severe acute respiratory syndrome coronavirus 2 (SARS-CoV-2) nasopharyngeal swab done earlier came back positive. While in the ICU the patient was found to be hypotensive and started on norepinephrine with escalating doses. A bedside TTE showed a hyperdynamic left ventricle (LV) with turbulent flow across the aortic valve. Further measurements revealed a mean gradient of 50 mmHg, peak velocity of 4.6 m/sec, aortic valve area of 0.90 cm^2, and Doppler velocity index (DVI) of 0.20 consistent with severe AS. She rapidly deteriorated and eventually passed away within 48 hours of her initially presentation.

Epidemiology: Coronavirus-19 disease or COVID-19 refers to a viral disease syndrome caused by SARS-CoV-2. Since the onset of the first cluster of cases reported in Wuhan, China, in December 2019, the disease has spread all over the world leading to a global pandemic. There were an estimated 27,236,916 confirmed cases including 891,031 deaths globally reported by the World Health Organization (WHO) by September 8, 2020.

Valvular heart disease (VHD) consists of a host of different pathologies both acquired and congenital that lead to a myriad of hemodynamic sequelae, symptoms, and clinical presentations. The prevalence of some of these pathologies increases with increasing age. Among them, AS is the most prevalent VHD in industrialized nations that leads to a surgical or a catheter-directed intervention. However, overall, mitral regurgitation (MR) is the most common valvular disorder found in patients, especially those over the age of 75. In a study conducted in the UK-based community, the prevalence of VHD in patients over the age of 65 was estimated to be at 11%. As diagnostic modalities increase, the rates of VHD are only expected to get higher.

Among patients affected by COVID-19, elderly patients, who often have undiagnosed VHD, infected with SARS-CoV-2 tend to have more severe cases with higher mortality rates. Since the prevalence of VHD increases with increasing age, it is vital to understand the important hemodynamic sequelae of these orders among patients afflicted with COVID-19.

Pathophysiology: Numerous systemic manifestations of infection with SARS-CoV-2 were uncovered as the pandemic unfolded globally. Some of these included, but were not limited to, neurologic, hematologic, cardiovascular, gastrointestinal, and renal involvement. There are two distinct ways SARS-CoV-2 can cause cardiovascular insults. They include the direct mechanism, which involves viral infiltration into myocardial tissue, resulting in cardiomyocyte death and inflammation, and an indirect mechanism that involves cardiac stress due to respiratory failure or hypoxemia along with its various hemodynamic consequences and cardiac inflammation secondary to severe systemic hyperinflammation.

While the mechanism in various VHDs revolves around abnormal flow through a pathologic valve, and its accompanying hemodynamic and structural consequences, in the subsequent section we will briefly explain the pathophysiologic mechanism in each valvular disorder and the possible effect of COVID-19 infection. Although literature exploring the pathophysiologic mechanism and resulting hemodynamic consequences of COVID-19 infections in patients with various VHDs are currently lacking, our explanation reflects the reasonable extrapolation of the common similar conditions and their consequences in patients with these disorders.

In patients with AS, the increasing resistance of flow from the LV into the aorta at the level of the aortic valve is most commonly from calcific degeneration of a normal trileaflet valve, rheumatic involvement, or calcification of a congenitally abnormal valve (bicuspid aortic valve). What initially starts as a compensatory mechanism to overcome the increasing resistance, leads to progressive LV remodeling in the form of hypertrophy and diastolic dysfunction that eventually leads to many of the myriad of symptoms including chest pain, shortness of breath, and syncope. On the other hand, in aortic regurgitation (AR), because of the improperly coapting valve leaflets, the blood regurgitates back into the LV causing a state of volume overload, eventually leading to eccentric hypertrophy and LV cavity dilation. In an attempt to keep up with these changes, the LV remodeling leads to a cascade of maladaptive responses that lead to its eventual failure and the various symptoms associated with it. Infection with SARS-CoV-2 may lead to a systemic inflammatory response that may cause profound vasodilation, and with it a reduced systemic vascular resistance. The selection of vasopressor in such patients may become tricky.

The pathophysiology in patients with MR revolves around a complex dynamic interplay between the abnormal forward and backward flow that creates deranged hemodynamics and produces varying signs and symptoms. Although patients with mild to moderate MR are initially well compensated, severe or sudden MR leads to significant LV volume overload beyond the capacities of compensation. This culminates in LV dilation along with systolic failure and worsened backflow into the traditionally low-pressure left atrium (LA), predisposing patients to the development of pulmonary edema. Patients who have been asymptomatic or minimally asymptomatic may be tipped into frank pulmonary edema from the various metabolic derangements that accompany SAR-CoV-2 infection. Similarly, in patients with mitral stenosis (MS), systemic changes that accompany COVID-19 infection, including tachycardia, increased cardiac output, and development of atrial fibrillation (AF), may cause worsening impediment to the normal transmitral flow of blood from LA to LV, leading to elevated LA pressures and thus pulmonary edema. (1-6)

DIAGNOSTICS

Symptomatology and appreciating classic signs associated with some of the VHDs may become challenging given that some patients are attached to multiple therapeutic machines like ventilators. Dyspnea and chest pain, especially in the setting of COVID-19 infection, may pose an extremely challenging clinical conundrum of whether the symptoms originate from COVID-19 per se or represent VHD manifesting in the setting of metabolic derangement from the infection.

The utility of inflammatory markers such as D-dimer, interleukin (IL)-6, ferritin, and lactate dehydrogenase (LDH) may aid in pointing to a rather severe case of COVID rather than VHD, even if severe VHD by itself does not lead to elevated levels of inflammatory markers. Given the nonspecific nature of these markers, they may not be completely applicable in a host of different clinical scenarios (e.g., bacterial sepsis complicating presentation). Chest X-ray, while an important initial and conveniently available tool, is not very specific when it comes to diagnosing valvular disorders.

Straightening of the left border of the heart or the so called "double-density" signs associated with MS, albeit rare, may aid in diagnosing specific valvular disorders. The presence of prosthetic valves, when history is not very clear, may also be appreciated on chest X-ray.

Echocardiography continues to remain an indispensable tool in the evaluation of patients with COVID-19 suspected to have VHD. Not only is it an invaluable resource in diagnosis of these conditions, but it also helps in elucidating the hemodynamic consequences occurring in these patients, given the widespread systemic manifestation resulting from COVID-19 infection. A bedside point-of-care ultrasound (POCUS) is the most commonly used initial strategy to gather preliminary information given the rapidity with which it can be performed. This should be followed by a formal TTE with a dedicated scanning protocol to obtain more detailed information. Echocardiography remains the most important diagnostic test in understanding valve structure and function in suspected cases as it is cheap, easy to perform, and readily available. Although it can be difficult to obtain images of satisfactory quality in certain patients (e.g., obese, mechanically ventilated, those with chronic obstructive pulmonary disease [COPD]), using Doppler to obtain gradients across valves can still provide sufficient clinical information for the management of critically ill patients.

Invasive testing finds limited utility as it risks significant exposure and contamination. Although TEE can be used to provide more detailed information about valvular pathologies, the application of such a modality in patients with active COVID-19 infection carries a significant risk of exposure to healthcare professionals due to potential aerosolization. It should only be pursued after understanding the risk-benefit assessment and if performing the test would meaningfully add to a patient's care.

Treatment: At the moment there are no evidence-based guidelines available on the management of VHD in patients with confirmed COVID-19 infection. Based on the European Society of Cardiology's (ESC) guidance on the management of cardiovascular diseases during the COVID-19 pandemic, we recommend a risk-stratified approach in managing patients with VHD. At the peak of the pandemic, given the divergence of all the resources and personnel available to care for patients battling COVID-19, low-risk patients with stable disease can be safely managed at home with aggressive monitoring of symptoms and telehealth-directed visits. High-risk patients, especially those who present in a state of decompensated disease process, may need emergent or urgent treatment for a specific valvular disorder.

A heart team approach involving holistic assessment of patients, including their symptoms, laboratory makers, and imaging findings, should be undertaken by a dedicated team of cardiologists, interventional cardiologists, and cardiothoracic surgeons to stratify patient risk. This helps in determining the necessity and degree of interventions and if they are required at all.

Patients with mild to moderate and severe VHD, but with minimal symptoms, should be managed with frequent telehealth visits focused on symptom assessment. Severe symptoms, on the other hand, merit a time-sensitive approach. Although medical therapy in patients with VHD and COVID-19 remains the cornerstone therapy, surgical interventions may be considered under special circumstances. For example, in a patient with AS syncope, New York Health Association (NYHA) Class III/IV symptoms, or angina, higher mean gradients (>50 mmHg) and peak velocities (>5 m/sec) on TTE would warrant urgent need for intervention. Similarly, in patients with decompensated disease with significant hemodynamic compromise precipitated from COVID, a trial of specific minimally invasive interventions could be considered within the framework of a heart team discussion. Physicians, however, should have a careful discussion about the risk and benefits of procedures with patients and family. Being frequently associated with systemic thrombosis, patients with COVID-19 infection considered for invasive procedures like transcatheter aortic valve replacement (TAVR) or surgical aortic valve replacement (SAVR) should be carefully monitored for the development of such complications. The futility of interventions and procedures among patients expected to have poor prognoses warrants important consideration and rationale, and this should be explained to these patients' families.

Therapeutics: As discussed above, the mainstay treatment for all VHDs tends to revolve around medical therapy, such as blood pressure and heart rate control and decongestion via diuresis. An important aspect of this also should focus on treatment of the primary offending condition, namely the various systemic manifestations of COVID-19. This section focuses on the various therapeutic interventions catered to each valvular disorder.

Decompensated AS patients, especially when medical management fails to show improvements, should be considered for emergent interventions. Balloon valvuloplasty (BAV) or TAVR/transcatheter aortic valve implantation (TAVI) can be a last resort. SAVR is frequently not a conducive option in such patients given their high risk, as assessed from various risk score calculators like the Society of Thoracic Surgeons (STS) score or EuroSCORE. BAV may be considered in selected acutely decompensated patients with favorable anatomy as a bridge to a more definitive intervention (TAVR/SAVR) at a later stage when they are hemodynamically more stable.

Selection of vasopressor agents in patients with cardiogenic and septic shock merits consideration of pathophysiology associated with AR. Dobutamine with its inotropic and chronotropic response and relative absence of vasoconstriction may be a suitable choice since tachycardia offers a favorable profile by shortening diastole and reducing time for regurgitation. TAVR can be a possibility if the aortic and valvular anatomy permits. However, like all other valvular pathologies considered for intervention, risk-benefit assessment along with feasibility and futility should be given due importance. (1-6)

Patients with stable primary and secondary MR with minimal or no symptoms can be managed with careful monitoring with optimal medical management, like goal-directed medical therapy for ischemic and nonischemic cardiomyopathies provided there are no contraindications like usage of afterload-reducing agents with septic shock. Patients who present with decompensated symptoms in the setting of acute primary MR (e.g., chordae rupture) and secondary MR not responding to medical management should be considered for transcatheter mitral edge-to-edge repair. However these procedures are frequently carried out under the guidance of

TEE, which predisposes operators and TEE operators to significant exposure.

Medical therapy remains our initial approach for decompensated heart failure symptoms. Diuretic therapy along with rate control, especially with AF, remains the mainstay. A beta blocker, with an added advantage of reducing cardiac output in addition to curbing tachycardia, which frequently occurs in the setting of infection with SARS-CoV-2, can be a useful agent. Patients with COVID-19 and MS who develop AF should be anticoagulated with heparin, vitamin K antagonist (Coumadin), or low-molecular-weight heparin (Lovenox). Direct-acting (novel) oral anticoagulants should be avoided as they have not been studied extensively in valvular AF. [1-6] Percutaneous balloon valvotomy may be considered in selected patients in whom medical management has failed and the patient continues to be symptomatic with evidence of pulmonary edema, provided the anatomy is feasible and there are no LA/LV clots or presence of more than mild MR (Figure 6-1).

KEY POINTS

- Appreciating classic signs and symptoms to diagnose specific VHD in patients with COVID-19 may not be easy because patients often need invasive therapies like mechanical ventilation.
- Echocardiography continues to remain an indispensable tool in the evaluation of patients with COVID-19 suspected to have VHD.
- Patients mild to moderate and severe VHD but with minimal symptoms should be managed with frequent televisits focused on symptom assessment.
- Although medical therapy in patients with VHD and COVID-19 remains the cornerstone therapy, surgical interventions may be considered under special circumstances under the framework of a heart team discussion.
- Futility of interventions/procedures among patients expected to have poor outcomes should warrant consideration. Decisions to proceed or avoid such procedures/intervention should be thoroughly discussed with patients and families.

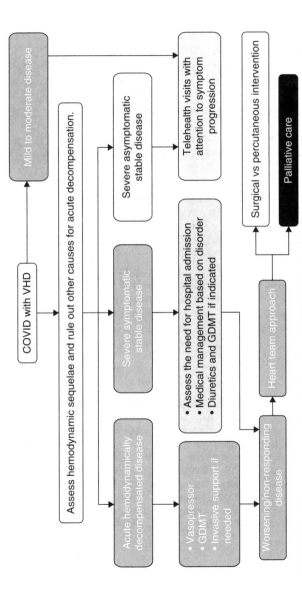

FIGURE 6-1 **Algorithm for management of valvular heart disease (VHD) in COVID patients.** GDMT, guideline-directed medical therapy.

PATIENT EDUCATION

What are valvular heart disorders?

Valvular heart disorders are a group of conditions that lead to abnormal blood flow through an abnormal heart valve. There are four valves in the heart: mitral, aortic, pulmonic, and tricuspid. The abnormal blood flow can lead to characteristic symptoms like shortness of breath, lightheadedness, falls, chest pain, and reduced exercise capacity.

Can having COVID-19 or getting infected with SARS-CoV-2 affect my VHD?

COVID-19 could potentially cause serious manifestation of VHD and worsen the symptoms. If you are diagnosed with COVID-19 and suffer from a VHD, please talk to your physicians for more information. If you do experience symptoms like shortness of breath, palpitations, loss of consciousness, and chest pain let your physician know.

Was scheduled for a procedure for my heart valve disorder. Should I postpone if I have been diagnosed with COVID-19?

Unless severe or emergent, as assessed by your physician, the procedure should be postponed with timely follow-up with your physician. If you do experience severe symptoms like chest pain and loss of consciousness, please alert your physician immediately.

References

1. World Health Organization. Pneumonia of unknown cause—China. Accessed January 5, 2020. https://www.who.int/csr/don/05-january-2020-pneumonia-of-unkown-cause-china/en/.

2. World Health Organization. WHO Coronavirus Disease (COVID-19) Dashboard. Accessed August 2020. https://covid19.who.int/.

3. Baumgartner H, Falk V, Bax JJ, et al. 2017 ESC/EACTS Guidelines for the management of valvular heart disease. *Eur Heart J.* 2017;38(36):2739-2791.

4. Nkomo VT, Gardin JM, Skelton TN, Gottdiener JS, Scott CG, Enriquez–Sarano M. Burden of valvular heart diseases: a population–based study. *Lancet.* 2006;368:1005-1011.

5. D'Arcy JL, Coffey S, Loudon MA, et al. Large–scale community echocardiographic screening reveals a major burden of undiagnosed valvular heart disease in older people: the OxVALVE Population Cohort Study. *Eur Heart J.* 2016;37:3515-3522.

6. Centers for Disease Control and Prevention (CDC). (Severe outcomes among patients with coronavirus disease 2019 (COVID-19): United States, February 12–March 16, 2020. *MMWR Morb Mortal Wkly Rep.* 2020;69(12): 343-346.

CHAPTER 7

COVID-19 and Myopericardial Disease

Niel Shah, Timothy J. Vittorio

CASE PRESENTATION

A Hispanic gentleman in his thirties presented to the emergency department with chest pain and fever. The chest pain was 7/10 in intensity, sharp in nature, intermittent, retrosternal in location, worsening with breathing movements, and radiating to the back. Additionally, he complained of subjective fever associated with chills and an episode of vomiting. The review of the system was negative otherwise. There was no significant past medical or surgical history. He did not have any family history of major cardiovascular disease. There was no recent travel or contact with known COVID-19 patients. The patient was a former smoker and stopped approximately 4 years ago. Last, he used to drink 2 pints of vodka every day but denied use of any other illicit drugs.

Vital signs were within normal limits, and the physical examination was unremarkable except for bilateral basilar dry rales on auscultation of the lungs. Laboratory tests were significant for leukocytosis (16.4/µL) with neutrophilic predominance, elevated C-reactive protein (CRP; 242 mg/L), elevated erythrocyte sedimentation rate (ESR; 76 mm/hr), elevated D-dimer (823 ng/mL), elevated lactate dehydrogenase (LDH; 475 units/L), elevated ferritin (676 ng/mL), and elevated troponin T levels (55 ng/L, normal ≤12 ng/L). Urine drug screen was negative. The initial 12-lead electrocardiogram (ECG) showed diffuse PR segment depression (Figure 7-1), which was suggestive of pericarditis in the setting of chest pain and subjective fever. Chest radiography (CXR) demonstrated multifocal pneumonia and

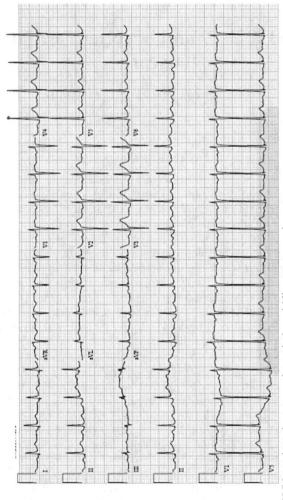

FIGURE 7-1 Initial ECG showing normal sinus rhythm and diffuse PR segment depression.

borderline enlarged cardiac silhouette likely secondary to cardiomegaly or pericardial fluid. A computed tomography (CT) scan of the chest with contrast excluded pulmonary embolism and showed normal heart and pericardium. Rapid influenza and COVID-19 real-time reverse-transcriptase polymerase chain reaction (rRT-PCR) testing were negative. Repeat troponin was trending upward (63 ng/L), so the patient was admitted in the coronary care unit (CCU) for suspected myopericarditis.

Anti-inflammatory therapy with colchicine and ibuprofen was begun for myopericarditis. The patient was started on broad-spectrum antibiotics empirically. He was maintained on droplet and contact isolation for COVID-19 as suspicion was high despite one negative COVID-19 rRT-PCR test. However, he was found to have positive antibodies for COVID-19 (anti–SARS-CoV-2 IgG/IgM reactive antibodies). Therefore, a provisional diagnosis of COVID-19 myopericarditis was made. The repeat COVID-19 rRT-PCR test was negative again. Due to suggested evidence of worsening outcome in COVID-19 patients with use of nonsteroidal anti-inflammatory drugs (NSAIDs), ibuprofen was discontinued. Instead, the patient was changed to oral prednisone and continued on colchicine for treatment. Transthoracic echocardiogram (TTE) revealed a left ventricular ejection fraction (LVEF) of 47%, eccentric left ventricular hypertrophy (LVH) with global LV wall motion abnormality, mild pulmonary hypertension, and no evidence of pericardial effusion. Based on these findings, low doses of angiotensin-converting enzyme inhibition (ACE-I) and β-adrenoceptor blockade (beta blocker) were begun for LV systolic dysfunction. During the hospital course, he became hypoxemic and required supplemental oxygen via nasal cannula. Moreover, he developed new-onset paroxysmal atrial fibrillation (PAF) (Figure 7-2) and was started on anticoagulation while continuing low dose beta-blockade.

The clinical symptoms improved with treatment. During the hospital course, inflammatory markers and cardiac troponin levels were monitored and continued to decline. There was no evidence for other infectious disease or underlying autoimmune disorder. A repeat TTE was unchanged. At the time of hospital discharge, he remained in normal sinus rhythm (NSR), but anticoagulation was continued until resolution of the myopericarditis. An outpatient

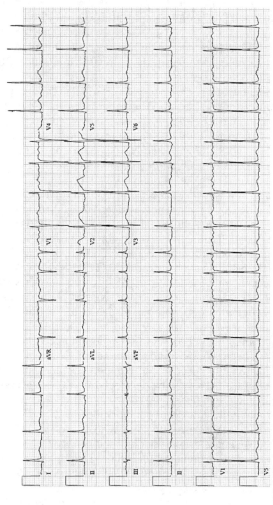

FIGURE 7-2 ECG showing new-onset atrial fibrillation.

tapering schedule was arranged for colchicine and prednisone treatment. After weaning the anti-inflammatory therapy, elective cardiac magnetic resonance imaging (cMRI) was planned.

INTRODUCTION AND EPIDEMIOLOGY

COVID-19 has several adverse effects on the cardiovascular system. Cardiac injury with troponin leak is associated with increased mortality in COVID-19, and its clinical and radiographic features are difficult to distinguish from those of heart failure (HF). Cardiac involvement may occur with COVID-19 even without respiratory tract signs and symptoms of infection. Viral infection has been widely described as one of the most common infectious causes of myopericardial diseases, such as, coxsackie, enterovirus, herpes simplex, cytomegalovirus, H1N1, respiratory syncytial virus, parvovirus B19, influenza, varicella, HIV, rubella, echovirus, and hepatitis B and C. The data about cardiac involvement as a complication of SARS-CoV-2 infection remain limited. There have been reported cases of myocarditis, myopericarditis (perimyocarditis), pericarditis, pericardial effusion, and cardiac tamponade in COVID-19 patients. Myocarditis results in focal or global myocardial inflammation, necrosis, and eventually LV systolic dysfunction. The prevalence of myopericardial diseases among COVID-19 patients is unclear. It has been reported that that up to 7% of COVID-19–related deaths were attributable to myocarditis. However, this was based on assumption and not on confirmatory diagnosis of myocarditis; thus, it may be an overestimate.

A significant number of patients admitted to the hospital with COVID-19 have an elevated serum troponin level, which is associated with an adverse outcome. Elevated troponin levels could result from various mechanisms or a combination of various mechanisms, such as right ventricular strain due to lung involvement and/or pulmonary emboli, a type 2 myocardial infarction due to hypoxemia or secondary to a systemic inflammatory response, or direct myocardial injury or inflammation causing myocarditis. A study was conducted on COVID-19-positive patients with elevated serum high-sensitivity troponin T (hsTnT) due to uncertain etiology and who underwent cardiac MRI. This study showed high incidence of myocarditis

(13 of 29 patients) and lower incidence of pericardial effusion (2 of 29) in such patients. The results of the study also showed a diagnosis of myocarditis in 1%-2% of the total number of rRT-PCR-positive patients and pericardial effusion diagnosed in approximately 10% of patients with COVID-19 myocarditis. Another study from Germany included a cohort of 100 patients who were recently recovered from COVID-19 and showed that 60% of patients had evidence of myocardial inflammation. Of those 60%, 70% had a detectable hsTnT (>3 pg/mL), whereas 5% had an hsTnT raised above the reference range (>13.9 pg/mL). On the other hand, about 20% of patients had a pericardial effusion >1 cm. In one meta-analysis approximately 5% of patients with COVID-19 who underwent CT of the chest had a detectable pericardial effusion.

Pathophysiology: Patients with previous cardiac disease and/or a structurally abnormal heart may be at increased risk of developing COVID-19 myopericarditis and cardiac tamponade. The definite mechanism of SARS-CoV-2-induced cardiac injury is unknown, but there are a few different possible theories:

1. Cytokine storm due to dysregulated but exaggerated immune response, which leads to increased vascular permeability, cell apoptosis, suboptimal T-cell and antibody responses, and acute respiratory distress syndrome (ARDS). Elevated levels of inflammatory markers have been seen in COVID-19 patients and a concomitant rise in cardiac biomarkers have been reported, which supports the cytokine release syndrome hypothesis. Interleukin (IL)-6 seems to be the central mediator of the cytokine storm, in which it promotes the proinflammatory responses from T lymphocytes. This process causes T-lymphocyte activation and a further release of inflammatory cytokines, which stimulate more T lymphocytes, leading to a positive feedback loop of immune activation and eventually myocardial damage. Cardiotropism of the T lymphocytes possibly arises from interaction between heart-produced hepatocyte growth factor (HGF) and c-Met, which is an HGF receptor on naive T lymphocytes.

2. Hypoxia secondary to SARS-CoV-2 ARDS, which can lead to inflammation, cell injury, and subsequent cardiac damage. It causes increased intracellular calcium deposition and apoptosis.

3. Direct injury by viral replication. One study reported the concurrent presence of a high SARS-CoV-2 viral load in patients with fulminant myocarditis. However, autopsies of COVID-19 patients revealed mononuclear cell inflammatory infiltrates without viral inclusions.

4. Angiotensin-converting enzyme 2 (ACE2)-mediated direct myocardial involvement. SARS-CoV-2 enters human cells by binding its spike protein to the membrane protein ACE2. ACE2 can be found on the ciliated columnar epithelial cells of the respiratory tract, type II pneumocytes, and cardiomyocytes. Therefore, it is possible that SARS-CoV-2 infects the human heart, especially in case of HF as ACE2 is upregulated, although the presence of viral receptors does not always predict tropism.

Clinical Features: Clinical presentation of COVID-19 myocarditis or myopericardial diseases varies and ranges from asymptomatic to cardiogenic shock. Some patients may present with relatively mild symptoms, such as fatigue and dyspnea. Others may present with chest discomfort with rest and/or exertion. Many patients deteriorate quickly and show symptoms of sinus tachycardia and acute HF with cardiogenic shock. In such severe cases, patients may present with signs of right-sided HF, which include peripheral edema, elevated jugular venous pressure, and right upper quadrant abdominal discomfort. The 12-lead ECG abnormalities observed in myocarditis might include new-onset bundle branch block, QTc interval prolongation, pseudoinfarction patterns, premature ventricular complexes and brady/tachyarrhythmias, and varying degrees of atrioventricular nodal block.

Patients with COVID-19 pericarditis may present with a variety of nonspecific signs and symptoms. The major clinical manifestations of acute pericarditis include fever, leukocytosis, chest discomfort, pericardial friction rub, 12-lead ECG changes, and possible pericardial effusion, which might lead to cardiac tamponade. These clinical manifestations sometimes precede the COVID-19 respiratory or gastrointestinal symptoms. Chest discomfort is usually sharp and pleuritic, which improves by sitting up and leaning forward. A pericardial friction rub is a superficial scratchy or squeaking sound that can be best heard with the diaphragm of the stethoscope over the left lower sternal border. The common 12-lead ECG changes in such patients include widespread concave ST segment elevation or PR segment depression. In some COVID-19 patients, pericarditis may lead to pericardial effusion or cardiac tamponade. Patients with cardiac tamponade show similar clinical presentations as seen in obstructive shock. Clinical findings commonly associated with cardiac tamponade include hypotension, sinus tachycardia, pulsus paradoxus, elevated jugular venous pressure, and muffled heart sounds. The combination of hypotension, elevated jugular venous pressure, and muffled heart sounds is known as Beck's triad. In cardiac tamponade patients, the 12-lead ECG may show low-voltage QRS complexes with electrical alternans, the latter resulting from the pendulum phenomenon.

Diagnosis: COVID-19–related myopericardial diseases can be suspected based on appropriate history including clinical presentation, travel history or exposure to sick contacts, and detailed physical examination and laboratory tests including COVID-19 rRT-PCR and inflammatory and cardiac markers. The 12-lead ECG and TTE findings may help further in making an appropriate diagnosis. Myocarditis is often suspected in patients presenting with chest discomfort after an influenza-like syndrome. There is usually clinical evidence suggesting an acute coronary syndrome (ACS) on 12-lead ECG or laboratory testing or with evidence of LV wall motion abnormalities without evidence of obstructive coronary artery disease as demonstrated by selective coronary angiography. Laboratory tests in myocarditis patients usually show elevated levels of lactate and other inflammatory markers, including CRP, ESR, and ferritin. These levels are usually increased in sepsis as well. It is especially important to distinguish fulminant myocarditis from sepsis because fluid resuscitation, which is a common practice in patients with sepsis, exacerbates fulminant myocarditis. Furthermore, it is advisable to test patients for baseline cardiac biomarkers, such as cardiac troponin and N-terminal pro–B-type natriuretic peptide (NT-proBNP) on hospital admission as these levels are elevated in myocarditis due to the acute myocardial injury, dysfunction, and possible ventricular dilation. In contrast, a negative troponin result cannot exclude myocarditis, particularly for atypical forms such as giant cell myocarditis or for those patients in the chronic phase. On the other hand, negative serial cardiac troponin levels are still helpful in the acute phase and make the diagnosis of acute myocarditis unlikely.

Additionally, cMRI, endomyocardial biopsy (EMB), or pericardial fluid analysis further help in confirming the diagnosis of COVID-19–related myopericardial diseases. The gold standard for the diagnosis of myocarditis is histological examination of the myocardium by EMB. However, a diagnosis of myocarditis can be made in the absence of EMB evidence, which requires an appropriate clinical syndrome along with evidence of myocardial edema, nonischemic late enhancement, and high T2 signaling on cMRI. EMB in patients with COVID-19 is not always possible due to limitations, such as critical illness, therefore, it is too unstable to transfer the patient to the cardiac catheterization laboratory or infection control measures prevent infected patients from being moved through the hospital for tests. However, tissue diagnoses of COVID-19 myocarditis, both pre- and postmortem have been reported in case series by confirming the presence of viral particles in the myocardium. Other cases of lymphocytic myocarditis in COVID-19 patients have been reported in Germany. A recent case series reported an analysis of cardiac tissue from 39 consecutive autopsies in elderly COVID-19 patients, which showed detection of SARS-CoV-2 RNA in the myocardium of 24 patients. However, there was no evidence of viral presence in cardiomyocytes and there was a lack of massive cell infiltration or evidence of cardiac necrosis; therefore, it was concluded that myocarditis was not present in those cases.

The role of pericardial fluid analysis in the diagnosis of COVID-19–related myopericardial diseases is controversial. There are case reports from Italy in which the pericardial fluid of one patient with COVID-19 tested positive for SARS-CoV-2 RNA; however, only one out of three viral genes was present, which suggested a low viral load. There are few more case reports of pericardial disease in COVID-19 patients, but in such case reports no comment has been made about whether the aspirated sample was infected or sterile. Finally, there are cases of pericardial disease in which pericardial fluid samples taken from COVID-19 patients were negative for SARS-CoV-2 (Table 7-1 and Figure 7-3).

TABLE 7-1 Diagnostic Findings Suggestive of COVID-19–Related Myopericardial Diseases

- Clinical presentation of chest discomfort after an influenza-like syndrome
- Elevated levels of lactate
- Elevated inflammatory markers, including CRP, ESR, and ferritin
- Elevated levels of cardiac biomarkers, such as cardiac troponin and NT-proBNP (negative troponin result cannot exclude myocarditis, but it can suggest the presence of a chronic variant of myocarditis)
- Evidence suggesting ACS on 12-lead ECG or LV wall motion abnormalities on 2D echocardiogram without evidence of obstructive coronary artery disease demonstrated by selective coronary angiography
- Evidence of myocardial edema, nonischemic late enhancement, and high T2 signaling on cMRI
- Pericardial fluid analysis is controversial because it may or may not show SARS-CoV-2 RNA
- Gold-standard for diagnosis of myocarditis is histological examination of the myocardium by EMB, which may show the presence of viral particles in the myocardium along with massive cell infiltration or evidence of cardiac necrosis

ACS, acute coronary syndrome; cMRI, cardiac magnetic resonance imaging; CRP, C-reactive protein; ECG, electrocardiogram; EMB, endomyocardial biopsy; ESR, erythrocyte sedimentation rate; LV, left ventricular; NT-proBNP, N-terminal pro–B-type natriuretic peptide.

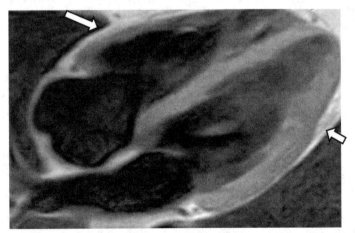

FIGURE 7-3 MRI showing the pericardial thickening in pericarditis.

Treatment: The best choice of pharmacological treatment for pericarditis in patients with COVID-19 needs more data and studies. NSAIDs are usually first line in all acute and recurring cases of pericarditis with no contraindications. However, a retrospective study performed in France showed that patients on NSAIDs for symptom control before hospitalization for pneumonia developed more severe forms of the disease and had longer hospitalization stays. Furthermore, worsening of symptoms in four COVID-19 patients was noted after receiving NSAIDs and this result was soon supported by the French Health Ministry. Published data have shown that ibuprofen increases the expression of ACE2 receptors. However, there is epidemiological evidence that does not allow the establishment of a causal link for the negative effect of ibuprofen in patients with COVID-19. Additionally, World Health Organization (WHO) and the American Food and Drug Administration (FDA) guidelines do not recommend interrupting the use of ibuprofen in symptomatic COVID-19 cases. Because of these controversial data and reports, the use of NSAIDs should be considered only after weighing the risk-benefit ratio in symptomatic COVID-19 patients.

Currently, colchicine has been increasingly used along with NSAIDs in treatment for acute and recurring pericarditis with excellent results; therefore, the use of colchicine should be considered in cases of COVID-19 patients with pericarditis. Regarding the use of colchicine in COVID-19 patients, at least eight studies are registered on clinicaltrials.gov for the evaluation of its effects in alleviating systemic and/or myocardial inflammation. Furthermore, two studies are already in progress: the Colchicine Coronavirus SARS-CoV-2 Trial (COLCORONA) and the ECLA PHRI COLCOVID Trial: Effects of Colchicine on Moderate/High-Risk Hospitalized COVID-19 Patients.

Corticosteroids are widely used in treatments for acute pericarditis because these drugs improve symptoms and reduce inflammatory markers. However, the COPE study showed that use of corticosteroids should be limited to cases of intolerance, contraindications, or failure of treatment with NSAIDs and colchicine due to an increased risk of recurrence. COVID-19 has been shown to have a unique pathophysiology with the state of hyperinflammation and cytokine storm; thus, the use of corticosteroids could be considered for COVID-19 pericarditis due to its anti-inflammatory properties.

However, the question remains: What is the ideal dose of corticosteroids in such patients? Potential risks of treatment with corticosteroids include risk of secondary infection and delay in viral clearance. Corticosteroids can be used in COVID-19 pericarditis patients as a substitute of NSAIDs with good results; however, more data are needed to support its use and to determine the best possible dose.

The management of COVID-19 myocarditis includes the use of immunomodulatory therapy, such as corticosteroids, intravenous immunoglobulin (IVIG), plasma exchange therapy, and cytokine inhibitors (tocilizumab). Antiviral agents such as remdesivir, supportive therapy such as mechanical ventilation, and cardiocirculatory-assist devices such as intra-aortic balloon pump counterpulsation are proved useful treatment modalities in patients with myocarditis. Ideally, treatment of myocarditis in COVID-19 patients should be modified based on the clinical presentation of each patient.

COMPLICATIONS

COVID-19 patients with pericarditis who develop cardiac tamponade should have pericardiocentesis performed without delay. Supportive treatment with fluid resuscitation and intravenous vasoactive therapy can prove effective while the patient is waiting for pericardiocentesis, but such supportive treatment should not be a substitute for the procedure. Some patients with COVID-19 pericarditis may develop pericardial effusion without hemodynamic compromise; these patients should undergo diagnostic pericardiocentesis to determine the underlying etiology, which may help in guiding further treatment. (1-7)

PROGNOSIS AND LONG-TERM FOLLOW-UP

During the COVID-19 pandemic, some COVID-19 patients with pericarditis were treated with chloroquine (CQ) and hydroxychloroquine (HCQ). However, there is no evidence on the efficacy and safety of these drugs. Patients with COVID-19 usually present with systemic inflammation and many patients develop concurrent myocarditis, which can lead to ventricular arrhythmias. HCQ is known for increasing the QTc interval, and increasing the risk of ventricular arrhythmias in such patients (Figure 7-4).

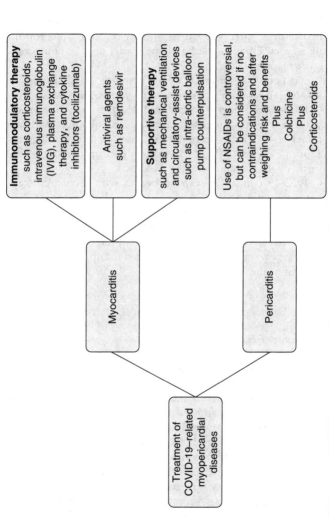

FIGURE 7-4 **Treatment of COVID-19–related myopericardial diseases.** NSAIDs, nonsteroidal anti-inflammatory drugs.

KEY POINTS

- The cardiac involvement in COVID-19 may be in the form of myocarditis, myopericarditis (perimyocarditis), pericarditis, pericardial effusion, cardiac tamponade, or a combination of more than one.
- Clinical presentation of COVID-19 myopericardial diseases varies and ranges from no symptoms to cardiogenic shock.
- COVID-19–related myopericardial diseases can be suspected with proper history taking, physical examination, and laboratory tests, which can be further supported by findings on a 12-lead ECG and TTE. EMB, cMRI, or pericardial fluid analysis further help in confirming the diagnosis.
- COVID-19 pericarditis can be treated with a combination of colchicine and NSAIDs, but the use of NSAIDs in COVID-19 patients is controversial, as some reports suggested worsening of symptoms with the use of NSAIDs in such patients. Corticosteroids are the alternative drugs and can be used with good results; however, more data are needed to support its use and to determine the best possible dosage.

PATIENT EDUCATION

What is myopericarditis?

It is the inflammation of the pericardium (sac around the heart), which can irritate the cardiac muscle and cause abnormal heart rhythm and symptoms such as chest pain and shortness of breath. The treatment is mainly pain medication and use of anti-inflammatory medications.

Can COVID-19 cause pericarditis?

Pericarditis can be observed in COVID-19-affected patients. It presents as chest pain that increases when laying flat and decreases with leaning forward. The symptoms can start at the time of onset of COVID-19 symptoms or it can start postinfection in the recovery phase. The symptoms may last for 4 weeks and can recur at any time depending on the extent of involvement of the pericardium.

Should I seek help if I have pericarditis?
Earlier detection and initiation of therapy will not only provide relief of symptoms but also help to avoid future complications and chances of recurrence. So it is important to seek an expert's assistance when symptoms are present.

References

1. Driggin E, Madhavan MV, Bikdeli B, et al. Cardiovascular considerations for patients, health care workers, and health systems during the coronavirus disease 2019 (COVID-19) pandemic. *J Am Coll Cardiol.* 2020;75:2352-2371.

2. Knight DS, Kotecha T, Razvi Y, et al. COVID-19: myocardial injury in survivors. *Circulation.* 2020;142:1120-1122.

3. Puntmann VO, Carerj ML, Wieters I, et al. Outcomes of cardiovascular magnetic resonance imaging in patients recently recovered from coronavirus disease 2019 (COVID-19). *JAMA Cardiol.* 2020;5(11):1265-1273.

4. Bao C, Liu X, Zhang H, Li Y, Liu J. Coronavirus disease 2019 (COVID-19) CT findings: a systematic review and meta-analysis. *J Am Coll Radiol.* 2020;17:701-709.

5. Lindner D, Fitzek A, Brauninger H, et al. Association of cardiac infection with SARS-CoV-2 in confirmed COVID-19 autopsy cases. *JAMA Cardiol.* 2020;5(11):1281-1285.

6. Farina A, Uccello G, Spreafico M, Bassanelli G, Savonitto S. SARS-CoV-2 detection in the pericardial fluid of a patient with cardiac tamponade. *Eur J Intern Med.* 2020;76:100-101.

7. Khatri A, Wallach F. Coronavirus disease 2019 (Covid-19) presenting as purulent fulminant myopericarditis and cardiac tamponade: A case report and literature review. *Heart Lung.* 2020;49(6):858-863.

CHAPTER 8

COVID-19 and Hypertension

Fareeha Alavi, Hitesh Gurjar

CASE PRESENTATION

A 76-year-old male with a medical history of diabetes and hypertension was brought to the emergency department (ED) by ambulance, with complaint of generalized weakness and mechanical fall. Patient was found on the ground on emergency medical services (EMS) arrival and was hypoxic to 89% on room air, which improved with 2 L of oxygen. As per patient, he had a positive COVID-19 test 1 week prior.

His initial symptoms were dry cough, worsening anorexia, worsening of generalized weakness, and lightheadedness for 1 week. Home medications included losartan and amlodipine. In the ED, his blood pressure (BP) was noted to be 185/95 mmHg, heart rate of 85 beats/min, afebrile, and oxygen saturation of 98% on 2 L nasal cannula. His physical examination showed bibasilar crackles on chest exam. Electrocardiogram (ECG) was unremarkable. Computed tomography (CT) of the head did not show any acute findings, and chest X-ray showed multifocal pneumonia. Laboratory tests showed an elevated inflammatory marker (see Table 8-1). He was started on ceftriaxone, azithromycin, and remdesivir. His BP was persistently elevated, and he was started on intravenous labetalol. He was transferred to the coronary care unit. Later he started to improve and was transitioned to oral antihypertensive medications. He completed antibiotics for 5 days and reported feeling better and was discharged home.

Epidemiology: As per definition based on the American College of Cardiology and American Heart Association guidelines released in

TABLE 8-1 Inflammatory Markers

Lactate dehydrogenase	1037>>528>>564
C-reactive protein	42.56>>127.47>>62.48
D-dimer	473>>521>>420
Ferritin	1179

2017, approximately 45 million adults in the United States are diagnosed with hypertension. The global burden of hypertension, which currently exceeds 1.4 billion people, is expected to exceed 1.6 billion adults by year 2025 and as of today hypertension remains the leading cause of death across the globe, especially in high-income countries.

The latest definition of hypertension uses the following BP cutoffs:

BP Category	SBP (mmHg)		DBP (mmHg)
Normal	<120	and	<80
Elevated	120-129	and	<80
Hypertension			
Stage 1	130-139	or	80-89
Stage 2	≥140	or	≥90

DBP, diastolic blood pressure; SBP, systolic blood pressure.

Patients with hypertension have associated modifiable and nonmodifiable risk factors. Among the modifiable risk factors, the common factors are cigarette smoking, diabetes mellitus, hypercholesterolemia, obesity, physical inactivity, and unhealthy diet. Relatively fixed risk factors are chronic kidney disease, family history of hypertension, increased age, low-socioeconomic status, male gender, obstructive sleep apnea, and psychosocial stress.

Hypertension and COVID-19. Today, the world is seriously affected by a global pandemic caused by SARS-CoV-2, which has caused huge loss of life, a significant economic crisis, and significant healthcare access problems. Due to various lockdown implementations and reduced mobility, various risk factors associated with hypertension are on the rise. Increased weight, indiscretion with dietary habits, physical inactivity, difficulty accessing medical healthcare, and fear of going to medical facilities have caused worsening factors contributing to hypertension. Whether these factors are going to play a major part in long-term outcomes remains to be seen. Especially worth mentioning is the fear of accessing healthcare facilities during the initial part of pandemic, during which hospitals witnessed a sudden decrease in the number of myocardial infarction patients coming to the hospital and undergoing primary percutaneous coronary interventions.

Hypertension is found to be common among patients hospitalized for COVID-19. Studies have shown that the prevalence of hypertension in patients with COVID-19 stands between 25% and 30%. However, whether it affects outcomes after admission due to COVID-19–related complications is neither clear nor confirmed. Because COVID-19 is known to cause worse outcomes in the elderly patient population, and prevalence of hypertension is also known to increase with age, the relationship may not be causal; it could be just an association due to age.

Pathophysiology:

Renin-angiotensinogen-aldosterone system. A great deal of interest arose in hypertension and COVID-19 association when it was discovered that angiotensin-converting enzyme 2 (ACE2) is an entry point for SARS-CoV-2 virus particles into the human body. This interaction between the renin-angiotensin-aldosterone system (RAAS) and SARS-CoV-2 has been an area of research lately.

The RAAS system is known to exert its effect on endothelial cell dysfunction, vascular remodeling, and hypertension.

Classic axis. Renin is produced by juxtaglomerular cells in the kidneys and is a protease that cleaves angiotensinogen produced by this liver. This leads to the production of angiotensin I (Ang 1), which is further converted to angiotensin II by ACE. ACE enzymes are most abundant in lungs; however, they are also found in tissues and vessels. Angiotensin II (Ang 2) exerts its effects through AT1 and AT2 receptors. Activation of AT1 receptors causes elevated BP, glucose intolerance, and atherosclerosis. AT2 receptor activation usually exerts protective effects by activating nitric oxide production and endothelial-dependent vasodilatation.

ACE2/Ang 1-7/MAS axis. Another important discovery is the production of heptapeptides Ang 1 through 7 (Ang 1-7) from both decapeptide Ang I and from Ang II. Ang 1-7 is produced from Ang I by endopeptidase and from Ang II by ACE homolog ACE2. This product, Ang 1-7, acts through the MAS pathway and exerts a multitude of protective effects in vascular biology.

A recent Prospective Urban Rural Epidemiology (PURE) study found increased levels of ACE2 associated with increased cardiovascular disease (CVD), possibly signifying increased downstream resistance to ACE2 effects, which increases the circulating levels of the enzyme.

Diagnostic Evaluation: Patients with hypertension are often asymptomatic; hence all persons older than 18 years of age should have their BP checked at least once and, if elevated, should undergo repeat measurements after an interval. Patients who are diagnosed with hypertension need careful assessment of risk factors including history of personal CVD, diabetes mellitus, dyslipidemia, chronic kidney disease, smoking status, diet, alcohol intake, physical activity, and psychosocial aspects. Family history of premature atherosclerosis, hypertension, diabetes, and hypercholesterolemia should also be evaluated. Patients with established hypertension should be assessed for target organ damage and assessed for cardiovascular risk. Patients who are young at diagnosis and have significant muscle weakness, arrythmias, flash pulmonary edema, palpitations, frequent headaches, snoring, and signs and symptoms suggestive of thyroid disease should be investigated for secondary causes of hypertension.

History and physical examination. Patients diagnosed with hypertension should undergo careful assessment for physical examination to look for signs of secondary hypertension and for target organ damage. The presence of carotid and renal bruits, enlarged kidney, enlarged thyroid gland, abdominal striae, radiofemoral delay, pedal edema, raised jugular venous pulse, and cardiac murmurs can hint at potential causes of hypertension or target organ damage.

Laboratory evaluation. Laboratory evaluation should include serum sodium, potassium, creatinine, lipid profile, fasting glucose; urine dipstick; and 12-lead ECGs. Based on clinical suspicion, additional laboratory investigations should be ordered including echocardiogram, carotid ultrasound, renal ultrasound, renal artery duplex, fundoscopic imaging, ankle brachial index, aldosterone-renin ratio, plasma free metanephrines, late-night salivary cortisol, urine albumin/creatinine ratio, uric acid levels, or liver function tests.

Therapeutic Options: Treatment of hypertension involves a multifactorial approach with involvement of the patient, physician, and social support. Lifestyle interventions are important and a necessary part of the multidisciplinary treatment of hypertension. Smoking cessation, regular exercise, weight reduction, low sodium intake, the Dietary Approach to Stop Hypertension (DASH) diet, and stress reduction are initial and necessary interventions.

Drug treatment includes primary agents, such as oral thiazide or thiazide-type diuretics, ACE inhibitors, angiotensin receptive blockers (ARBs), and calcium channel blockers (CCBs; dihydropyridines and nondihydropyridines). Secondary agents include loop diuretics, potassium-sparing diuretics, aldosterone antagonists, beta blockers (with cardioselective, vasodilatory, noncardioselective, intrinsic sympathetic activity, and combined α- and β-receptor activities), centrally acting alpha-2 agonists (clonidine, methyldopa), and directly acting drugs including hydralazine and minoxidil.

ACE inhibitors and COVID-19. ACE inhibitors and ARBs commonly used as antihypertensives are known to increase ACE2 levels. Because the ACE2 enzyme has also been found to be the receptor protein for SARS-CoV-2, concerns arose whether use of ACE inhibitors or ARBs causing increased levels of ACE2 could worsen COVID-19 infection by providing more entry points for SARS-CoV-2. However, large studies have failed to find any harmful effects of ACE inhibitors or ARBs in patients infected with SARS-CoV-2. So far, the consensus is to continue antihypertensives without any change in treatment regimes.

Aggressive need for BP control for hospitalized patients. Patients who are seriously ill and affected by COVID-19–related complications should be continued on antihypertensives. However, the decision to aggressively control BP should be weighed with anticipation of progression of COVID-19–related complications. If concerns of serious decompensation are anticipated, then BP goals should be liberalized, as the risk of developing hypotension in the short term would outweigh the benefits of tight BP control over the long term. (1-4)

Monitoring and Follow-Up:
Telehealth. Fear of being exposed to coronavirus has led to difficulties in accessing healthcare. Although public health measures are in effect, the concern remains significant. Telehealth provides the opportunity to provide continued medical care in these unprecedent times. It reduces the risk of exposure to both patient and healthcare providers. However, once concerns are raised and serious issues are anticipated, the patient should be appropriately advised for in-person appointments or to seek urgent in hospital care.

KEY POINTS

- Hypertension remains an important associated factor in patients developing a serious COVID-19 infection; however, in multivariate analyses it has not been shown to increase odd ratios of mortality.
- ACE homologue ACE2 is an important entry point for virus in the human body; however, ACE inhibitor or ARB use is not associated with any harmful effects or increased chances of infection, hence, treatment of hypertension should continue without any modifications.
- ACE2 and Ang 1-7 pathways acting through MAS pathways are increasingly recognized pathways exerting protective effects in vascular biology and serve as a counter-regulatory arm to proinflammatory- and fibrosis-generating pathways acting through AT1 receptors.

- Tighter in-hospital control of BP should be weighed with anticipation of developing hypotension and the need for ventilation in the short term.
- Telehealth is an important tool in providing continued healthcare services without risk of exposure to SARS-CoV-2.

PATIENT EDUCATION

I have hypertension and I heard from my friend and social media that I am at increased risk of complications? I am scared about it.

Although hypertension has been found to be quite common in patients with serious COVID-19 infections, whether it increases chances of getting serious infection or developing complications secondary to an infection is not established by research.

I have been exposed to a COVID-19 patient; should I change my antihypertensive medications?

Studies have refuted the initial concerns about use of antihypertensives like lisinopril and enalapril, which come under a group of antihypertensives called ACE inhibitors. Similarly, ARBs like losartan, valsartan, telmisartan, and so forth should be continued.

I am too scared to step out of my house. How can I contact my doctor?

Most hospitals and care providers are using telehealth. You can contact your hospital or care provider and schedule an appointment using telehealth. Your doctor will usually be able to call and assess you via a video call.

References

1. Whelton PK, Carey RM, Aronow WS, et al. 2017 ACC/AHA/AAPA/ABC/ACPM/AGS/APhA/ASH/ASPC/NMA/PCNA Guideline for the Prevention, Detection, Evaluation, and Management of High Blood Pressure in Adults: A Report of the American College of Cardiology/American Heart Association Task Force on Clinical Practice Guidelines. *Hypertension.* 2018;71(6):e13-e115.
2. Narula S, Yusuf S, Chong M, et al. Plasma ACE2 and risk of death or cardiometabolic diseases: a case-cohort analysis. *Lancet.* 2020;396(10256):968-976.

3. Donoghue M, Hsieh F, Baronas E, et al. A novel angiotensin-converting enzyme-related carboxypeptidase (ACE2) converts angiotensin I to angiotensin 1-9. *Circ Res.* 2000;87(5):E1-E9.
4. Santos RAS, Sampaio WO, Alzamora AC, et al. The ACE2/angiotensin-(1-7)/MAS axis of the renin-angiotensin system: focus on angiotensin-(1-7). *Physiol Rev.* 2018;98(1):505-553.

CHAPTER 9

COVID-19 and Cardiogenic Shock

Angel De La Cruz, Amandeep Singh

CASE PRESENTATION

The patient is a 61-year-old woman with medical history significant for hypertension, type 2 diabetes mellitus, hyperlipidemia, coronary artery disease, chronic kidney disease, and chronic obstructive pulmonary disease who presented to the hospital with complaints of chest pain and shortness of breath. When the patient arrived at the emergency department, she reported that the first symptom she experienced was shortness of breath. Shortness of breath started about 3 days before presentation with progressive worsening. Chest pain started 36 hours ago with gradual increase in intensity. Chest pain was described as left sided, 10/10, dull like, radiating to the epigastric area, and not improved with aspirin. The patient reported pain was worse with exertion. Symptoms were associated with mild dry cough, body aches, and fever. No runny nose, orthopnea, paroxysmal nocturnal dyspnea, palpitations, or lower extremity edema. She also denied abdominal pain, nausea, vomiting, and changes in bowel or bladder habits. The patient's husband had fever and cough for the last 2 weeks.

On physical exam, the patient seemed acutely ill and was noted to be short of breath. Initial vital signs recorded her to be febrile to 102°F, with a blood pressure of 92/56 mmHg, heart rate 102 beats/min, and respiratory rate 28 breaths/min. She was initially alert and responsive. Rales were heard in the bilateral lung fields. Cardiovascular examination was significant for tachycardia, S1 was normal, S2 was soft, S3 and S4 were heard, and a 2/6 systolic murmur was audible mostly in the aortic area without rub. Minutes after the first medical interaction the patient became pale and lethargic.

Electrocardiogram (ECG) showed sinus tachycardia and non-specific ST-T changes. Chest X-ray showed cardiomegaly and pulmonary hilum congestion along with peripheral opacities. The blood work results are shown in Table 9-1. White blood cell (WBC) count was decreased and a significant decrease in the lymphocyte percentage was noted. Thrombocytopenia, elevation in C-reactive protein

TABLE 9-1 Laboratory Data on Admission

Parameter	Result
WBC count	2.2×10^9/L
-Neutrophils	69%
-Lymphocytes	2.0%
-Eosinophils	12%
-Monocytes	17%
Hemoglobin	11.2 g/dL
Hematocrit	33.6%
Platelets	112×10^9/L
C-reactive protein	20.2 mg/dL
Troponin (HS)	92 ng/mL
Pro-BNP	2790 pg/mL
Sodium	141 mEq/L
Potassium	3.4 mEq/L
BUN	30 mg/dL
Creatinine	2.4 mg/dL
Aspartate aminotransferase	84 U/L
Alanine aminotransferase	78 U/L
D-dimer	510 ng/mL
Ferritin	240 ng/mL
Lactic acid	6.2 mg/dL

BUN, blood urea nitrogen, HS, high sensitivity; pro-BNP, pro-brain natriuretic peptide; WBC, white blood cells.

(CRP), troponin, pro-brain natriuretic peptide (BNP), lactic acid, and ferritin were found. Chemistry panel was suggestive of renal failure with mild elevation in the liver function tests. SARS-CoV-2 nasopharyngeal swab was sent.

Point-of-care echocardiogram was significant for severely decreased left ventricular contractility along with a mild amount of fluid in the pericardial space. The patient was taken to the catheterization lab, which did not reveal any significant obstructive coronary artery disease. Minutes after the procedure, her blood pressure dropped to 72/44 mmHg and the patient's limbs became cold. A cardiotonic agent was started. Corticosteroids were also started.

Computed tomography (CT) of the chest showed diffuse ground-glass opacities. SARS-CoV-2 nasopharyngeal swab came back positive. Her cardiotonic requirements were increasing significantly over the last 12 hours. Laboratory values showed increasing renal failure, ferritin, and CRP. Patient passed away within 36 hours of initial medical interaction.

DISCUSSION

Epidemiology: COVID-19 is caused by infection with the SARS-CoV-2. The principal target cells for the virus to infect are the epithelial cells of the respiratory tract, but viral RNA has also been found in other tissues, such as the cardiac tissue. Most patients with this condition remain asymptomatic, some can present with mild respiratory symptom, and few can have more severe presentations such as cardiogenic shock. Cardiovascular manifestations of COVID-19 are variable, and they may include arrhythmias, heart failure, and myocarditis. Data regarding the etiology, epidemiology, and management approach of cardiogenic shock in COVID-19 are limited at this time. To date, one of the most common described causes of cardiogenic shock in COVID-19 patients is acute coronary syndrome. About 50% of the patients that present to the hospital with ST-segment elevation myocardial infarction (STEMI), and test positive for SARS-CoV-2, develop cardiogenic shock, increasing mortality significantly in these patients. In the group of patients with STEMI, positive SARS-CoV-2 test, and cardiogenic shock, 75% die. However, it is important to note that during the peak of the pandemic, a 40% decrease in acute myocardial infarctions and delays in presentation to the hospitals have been reported. This fact may alter significantly the incidence of cardiogenic shock in patients positive for SARS-CoV-2. Because of delayed presentations, the incidence of acute myocardial infarctions with severe hemodynamic alterations have increased. In an Italian study analyzing data from intensive care units, the rate of myocardial infarction with complications, such as cardiogenic shock, increased during the first week after the initial lockdown. Data may vary from country to country. Numbers may vary now as patients start to come back to the hospitals in a timely manner. It is possible that the increased rate of cardiogenic shock related to myocardial infarction during the peak of the pandemic could be related to prolonged ischemia and progressive myocardial dysfunction due to delayed presentation.

Pathophysiology: Multiple causes can explain why patients with COVID-19 develop cardiogenic shock. The ones that have been more frequently described in the literature are acute fulminant myocarditis, stress-mediated cardiomyopathy, coronary artery thrombosis, and pulmonary thromboembolism. All of these may occur even in the absence of comorbid conditions. Because there are many possible etiologies of cardiogenic shock in COVID-19 patients, a thorough history, physical exam, and proper assessment of the lab data are needed to properly address the underlying condition.

COVID-19 can induce a systemic hypercoagulable state that may present as cardiogenic shock due to coronary thrombosis or pulmonary thromboembolism. The increased thromboembolic risk may also explain the risk of developing myocardial infarction, although the complete mechanism is not fully understood. Patients aged more than 65, with diabetes, hypertension, and/or dyslipidemia, are at increased risk.

Stress-related cardiomyopathy in patients infected with SARS-CoV-2 is likely related to adrenergic surge secondary to the inflammatory process, sepsis, hypoxemia, or myocardial infection with the virus of concern. A combination of factors is the most likely mechanism. Other mechanisms that may explain myocardial injury in patients with COVID-19 include elevated right ventricular afterload due to respiratory acidosis, and oxygen supply/demand mismatch.

In general, any inciting event that evolves into cardiogenic shock is characterized by profound depression of the cardiac contractility, which causes reduced cardiac output, leading to decreased blood pressure, which causes further coronary ischemia with concomitant further reduction in the myocardial contractility. Endothelial dysfunction could lead to increased risk of myocardial infarction and heart failure due to thrombosis, coagulopathy, and low nitric oxide levels. Release of tumor necrosis factors and various interleukins may account for the decreased adrenergic sensitivity and decreased contractility of the cardiac muscle, leading to death if not treated appropriately.

Diagnostic Modalities: There is no separate approach described for patients with cardiogenic shock and COVID-19. The same standard protocols used for any patient with cardiogenic shock are used. Initial protocol should include an ECG, chest radiography, laboratory tests (complete blood counts, complete metabolic panel, creatine kinase, troponin, pro-BNP, lactic acid, blood gas, and blood cultures). ECG can vary from sinus tachycardia, bigeminy, atrial arrhythmias, or significant ST-T changes. Performing early transthoracic echocardiography is crucial in all COVID patients with hypotension/cardiogenic shock to assess for left and right ventricle function, wall motion abnormalities, valvular abnormalities, and pericardial effusion. Coronary angiography and right-sided heart catheterizations may be appropriate based on clinical presentation. (1-3) If there is clinical suspicion for myocarditis, an endomyocardial biopsy can also be considered (Figure 9-1).

Therapeutics and Complications: Overall, the basic approach of management includes general routine measures, such as inotropes/vasopressors and mechanical ventilation, for cardiovascular and pulmonary support; systemic corticosteroids; and anticoagulation in certain cases. Corticosteroids are particularly useful in patients with myocarditis as they can reduce the infiltration of WBCs into the cardiac tissue, decreasing cardiac symptoms. In cases of acute coronary thrombosis, management should be directed toward percutaneous revascularization. An early invasive approach is usually recommended, but fibrinolysis can be considered in cases where

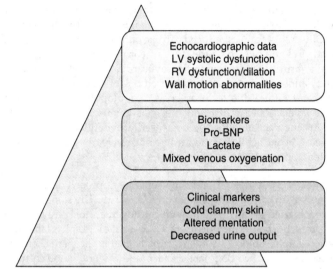

Echocardiographic data
LV systolic dysfunction
RV dysfunction/dilation
Wall motion abnormalities

Biomarkers
Pro-BNP
Lactate
Mixed venous oxygenation

Clinical markers
Cold clammy skin
Altered mentation
Decreased urine output

FIGURE 9-1 **Diagnostic algorithm in cardiogenic shock.**

percutaneous coronary intervention cannot be performed in a timely manner. In cases of pulmonary thromboembolism, management may also include thrombolysis or percutaneous management (in case thrombolysis is contraindicated). Patients who have an increasing pressor requirement or clinical deterioration should be evaluated for temporary mechanical circulatory support including venoarterial-extracorporeal membrane oxygenation (VA-ECMO) and percutaneous ventricular assist device. It is also key to manage the viral infection accordingly to provide comprehensive management.

In patients with the "wet and cold" presentation, the vasoactive agent of choice is norepinephrine; an inotropic agent can be added, but this should be assessed on a case-by-case basis. In patients with the "cold and dry-euvolemic" presentation, dopamine and norepinephrine can also be used, along with an inotropic agent (case-by-case consideration). (4-5) The hemodynamic effects of the most commonly used inotropes and inodilators are presented in Table 9-2.

TABLE 9-2 Hemodynamic Effects of the Most Common Inotropes and Inodilators Used in Cardiogenic Shock

Medication	Hemodynamic Effects
Dopamine	Increases cardiac output
Norepinephrine	Increases systemic vascular resistance and cardiac output
Phenylephrine	Increases systemic vascular resistance
Vasopressin	Increases systemic vascular resistance
Epinephrine	Increases systemic vascular resistance and cardiac output
Dobutamine	Increases cardiac output, decreases systemic vascular resistance
Milrinone	Increases cardiac output, decreases systemic vascular resistance
Isoproterenol	Increases cardiac output, decreases systemic vascular resistance

Cases when myocardial infarction is complicated with cardiogenic shock in the setting of COVID-19, the patient's recovery becomes more challenging. Therefore, constant monitoring and a proper surveillance strategy of the hemodynamics and lab data are important (Figure 9-2).

Constant monitoring of blood pressure, heart rate, respiratory rate, pulse oximetry, and temperature is the cornerstone in patients with cardiogenic shock. These patients should be managed in a critical care setting. Continuous monitoring of the arterial blood pressure and central venous pressure is also needed. A Swan-Ganz catheter for hemodynamic monitoring should be considered in cases complicated by cardiogenic shock. Periodical monitoring of the lactic acid and mixed venous oxygen saturation levels are appropriate to assess how effective the interventions have been in the patient under concern. Urine output should be monitored at least every 2 hours. If urine output is decreased, it is likely because of renal hypoperfusion, which is related to increased mortality. Furthermore, complete blood counts, electrolyte levels, markers of the liver and renal function tests, and lactate and coagulation studies should be done at least every 12 hours. Particularly, lactic acid levels have been described as important markers with prognostic value.

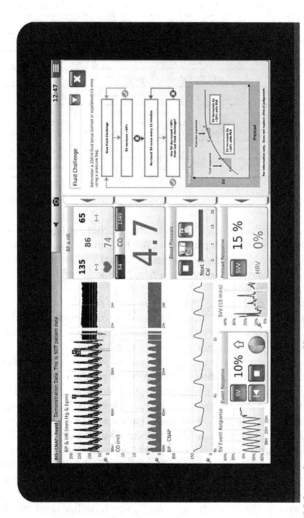

FIGURE 9-2 Hemodynamic monitor using an arterial line (LIDCO).

Prognosis and Long-Term Follow-Up: Patients that undergo percutaneous coronary intervention, without bleeding complications and no increased bleeding risk, should be continued on dual antiplatelet therapy. The medical team should be watchful for bleeding complications in these cases. The palliative care team should be on-board in patients with poor prognoses to have a complete interdisciplinary team taking care of the patients and supporting family members. Future directions in the management of COVID-19–related cardiogenic shock are geared not only toward management approaches but also toward monitoring and prognostic values that will provide a better understanding of this challenging condition (Figure 9-3).

KEY POINTS

- The main target cells for the SARS-CoV-2 to infect are the epithelial cells of the respiratory tract, but the virus may also infect other tissues, such as the cardiac tissue.
- Cardiovascular manifestations of COVID-19 are variable, and they may include arrhythmias, heart failure, and myocarditis. All of these may be complicated with cardiogenic shock.
- Mechanisms of COVID-19–mediated cardiogenic shock include the combination of a systemic hypercoagulable state, adrenergic surge secondary to the inflammatory process/sepsis/hypoxemia, and myocardial cell infection.
- In the group of patients with STEMI, positive SARS-CoV-2 test, and cardiogenic shock, mortality has been described to be around 75%.
- During the pandemic lockdown, because of delayed presentations, the incidence of acute myocardial infarctions with severe hemodynamic alterations increased. This mechanism is related to prolonged ischemia and progressive myocardial dysfunction.
- The same standard protocols used for any patient with cardiogenic shock are used in patients with COVID-19, along with isolation protocols. Initial protocol should include ECG, chest radiograph, lab data, coronary angiography, and in some cases endomyocardial biopsy. Constant monitoring of

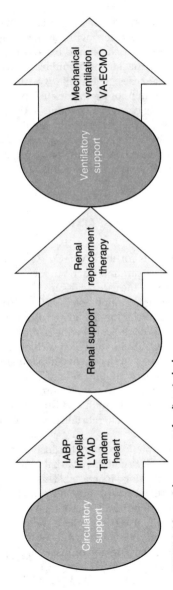

FIGURE 9-3 Sequential management of cardiogenic shock.

hemodynamic parameters is needed in these patients, who require a critical-care-unit level of care.

- Inotropes/vasopressors, mechanical ventilation, systemic corticosteroids, VA-ECMO, and implantable ventricular assist device should be considered. It is also key to manage the viral infection accordingly to provide comprehensive management.

PATIENT EDUCATION

What are symptoms of cardiogenic shock?

The most important component of patient education is to keep in mind that early presentation save lives! If respiratory symptoms, such as cough and shortness of breath, are accompanied by chest pain, fever, or lower extremity swelling, seeking immediate medical care is appropriate. The earlier the better so that a physician can plan accordingly and provide all the necessary measures in a timely manner.

COVID-19 is a disease caused by the novel coronavirus. Most patients infected with the virus will not get severely sick. It may cause shortness of breath, cough, fever, chills, weakness, headaches, sore throat, and absence of taste or smell. The majority of patients will improve within 2-3 weeks, but some patients will have severe symptoms and will need hospitalization. If you have symptoms it is appropriate to seek medical attention. If symptoms are not severe it is better to call your doctor before having an in-person visit.

In case you have more severe symptoms, or you think there is a medical emergency, call 9-1-1. This is especially important if you have chest pain or shortness of breath. Cardiogenic shock is a condition where, because the heart is not pumping blood effectively, all the organs in the body do not get sufficient blood supply and therefore do not work appropriately. It can also cause death. Cardiogenic shock can be seen in patients with COVID-19. When patients develop cardiogenic shock associated with COVID-19, doctors may consider providing therapies such as remdesivir or plasma exchange therapy to aid in fighting against the viral infection. They will also provide special medications to help keep the blood pressure within an appropriate range and to keep enough blood supply to the brain, heart, kidneys, liver, and other key organs. In that case, you will be hospitalized in a critical care unit.

How can I prevent cardiogenic shock?

Overall, at this time, the recommendation to prevent viral infection is to wear a face mask to prevent the spread of this deadly virus. Some recommendations that may help to maintain good overall health will also help to avoid cardiogenic shock: exercise regularly, avoid alcohol, do not smoke, decrease the ingestion of sugars in the diet, eat less saturated fats, and maintain a healthy weight. If comorbid conditions exist, such as hypertension and diabetes, appropriate management is needed because when uncontrolled, they may be associated with adverse cardiovascular outcomes in patients infected with COVID-19.

References

1. Sánchez-Recalde Á, Solano-López J, Miguelena-Hycka J, Martín-Pinacho JJ, Sanmartín M, Zamorano JL. COVID-19 and cardiogenic shock. Different cardiovascular presentations with high mortality. *Rev Esp Cardiol (Engl Ed)*. 2020;73(8):669-672.

2. Lauridsen MD, Butt JH, Østergaard L, et al. Incidence of acute myocardial infarction-related cardiogenic shock during corona virus disease 19 (COVID-19) pandemic. *Int J Cardiol Heart Vasc*. 2020;31:100659.

3. Chau VQ, Giustino G, Mahmood K, et al. Cardiogenic shock and hyperinflammatory syndrome in young males with COVID-19. *Circ Heart Fail*. 2020;13(10):e007485.

4. Tavazzi G, Pellegrini C, Maurelli M, et al. Myocardial localization of coronavirus in COVID-19 cardiogenic shock. *Eur J Heart Fail*. 2020;22(5):911-915.

5. Van Diepen S, Katz JN, Albert NM, et al. Contemporary management of cardiogenic shock: a scientific statement from the American Heart Association. *Circulation*. 2017;136(16):e232-e268.

CHAPTER 10

COVID-19 Management Strategies

Sᴀʀᴛʜᴀᴋ Kᴜʟsʜʀᴇsʜᴛʜᴀ,
Mᴜʜᴀᴍᴍᴀᴅ Hᴀssᴀɴ

CASE PRESENTATION

A 71-year-old Hispanic man with medical comorbidities of diabetes mellitus, hypertension, abnormal functioning bioprosthetic aortic valve (severe aortic stenosis), and chronic kidney disease was admitted with COVID-19 pneumonia confirmed with nasopharyngeal COVID-19 reverse-transcription-polymerase chain reaction (RT-PCR) test. The patient received tocilizumab, remdesivir and dexamethasone with marked signs of improvement. He was discharged home on a tapering dose of prednisone and home oxygen. He was readmitted 3 months later with fever and chills. His blood cultures grew methicillin-sensitive *Staphylococcus aureus*. He was started on intravenous antibiotics for 4 weeks but remained febrile with persistent bacteremia. An electrocardiogram showed third-degree heart block (Figure 10-1A). The patient underwent a transesophageal echocardiogram (TEE) for evaluation of endocarditis (Figure 10-1B). The TEE showed aortic valve vegetation with aortic root and aortomitral curtain thickening suspicious of abscess (Figure 10-1C). He underwent aortic root abscess drainage and implantation of a redo bioprosthetic aortic valve with transvenous pacemaker placement.

COVID-19 THERAPEUTICS

The management strategies of COVID-19 infection are controversial and still evolving. Physicians should be mindful of the pros and cons of therapeutics and their appropriateness in select

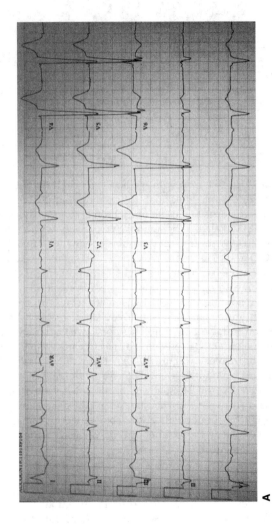

A

FIGURE 10-1 **(A)** ECG showing third-degree heart block. **(B)** TEE showed aortomitral curtain abscess. **(C)** Postoperative aortic valve.

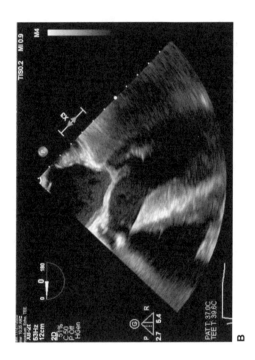

FIGURE 10-1 (Continued)

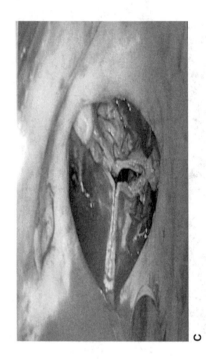

C

FIGURE 10-1 (*Continued*)

population groups. Immunization and development of antibodies against infection may have a promising future that is not yet known. The earlier data regarding the role of antibodies in COVID-19 infection showed that acquired immunity may have a protective role in avoiding disease and its complications, but the long-term effects beyond 6 months' duration remains elusive. Antibodies such as IgM and IgA are short-lived, lasting 2-4 weeks compared with antibody IgG that may last up to 6 months. Antibody titers at 6 months may have a role in predicting the immunity against the infection. Ongoing research will continue to prove the beneficial effects of antibodies in the long term and its system-based effectiveness. The cardiovascular effects of these immunization techniques are not clear.

Types of Immunization:

Active immunity. Active immunity in COVID-19 infection can be achieved using four strategies:

1. Whole virus. Whole virus in attenuated/killed form can trigger immunity. It can develop strong immunity but can cause disease in a weaker immune system. It requires cold chain for storage.
2. Protein subunit. A small subunit protein of virus is inoculated, which may generate immunity that can be weak or may not be completely protective.
3. Nucleic acid. Viral DNA/RNA is transferred to a human cell where it can generate antigen and antibodies with protective effects. It requires cold storage.
4. Viral vector. A nonpathogenic virus is introduced to create immunity in the body that can defend against actual viral infection.

Passive immunity. Convalescent plasma therapy has been approved by the US Food and Drug Administration (FDA) as an option for management of critically ill COVID-19 patients. It may have a beneficial role, but it has not been established as a cornerstone therapeutic for COVID-19 infection.

Available vaccines. Currently, there are around 165 different vaccines under development. These different vaccines utilize various mechanism such as mRNA, DNA, vectors, and inactivated and recombinant proteins to target the virus inside the human body. The primary aim for these vaccinations is to produce immunogenicity against COVID-19 virus.

Here are some of the major vaccines available and under development (Table 10-1).

1. Moderna Therapeutics (mRNA-1273)
   - In the COVE study phase 3 trial, more than 30,000 people greater than age 18 years were enrolled and has shown efficacy against COIVD-19 infection (94.1%).
   - The vaccine has received emergency use authorization by FDA.
   - The vaccine has shelf life of 7-30 days and can be stored at standard refrigeration temperatures.
   - Common side effects are injection site pain and erythema, fatigue, and myalgias. Long-term effects are unknown.
2. Pfizer (BNT162)
   - Joint venture between Pfizer and BioNTech (German biotech company).
   - The program is evaluating four different experimental vaccines that comprise unique variations of mRNA and target antigen.
   - Two vaccine prototypes are nucleoside modified RNA (modRNA), one is uridine containing (uRNA), and the last one has a self-amplifying mRNA (saRNA). Each of them is combined with a lipid nanoparticle (LNP) formulation.
   - Phase 3 trial enrolled above 43,000 subjects and has shown 95% efficacy against COVID-19 infection at 1 month.
   - Safety analysis showed one death from cardiac arrest and arteriosclerosis and one event of ventricular arrythmia.
3. University of Oxford (ChAdOx1 nCoV-19)
   - Based in the United Kingdom.
   - Phase 3 is being conducted in Brazil, South Africa, the United States, and India.
   - It is a viral vector vaccine using adenovirus.
   - The study enrolled 23,000 subjects with 90% efficacy.
   - Safety profile needs to be determined.

TABLE 10-1 Recent Data about COVID Vaccine

Vaccine Developing Company	Type of Vaccine	No. of Doses Needed	Efficacy (%)	Likely Emergency Use Authorization (EUA) Date	Storage Requirements	Status	Route of Administration
Pfizer BioNTech	Modified mRNA	2, 28 days apart	95	December 10, 2020	−94°F	Approved by the FDA	Intramuscular
Moderna-mRNA-1273	RNA	2, 28 days apart	94.5	December 10, 2020	36-46°F, for up to 30 days	Approved by the FDA	Intramuscular
Oxford-AstraZeneca	Viral vector	2, 28 days apart	90	Possibly January 2021, but unclear in the United States	36-46°F, for up to 6 months	Approved in UK	Intramuscular
Gamaleya (Sputnik V)	Viral vector	2	95	Unlikely to be used in the United States	-	Phase III trial	Intramuscular
Johnson & Johnson	Viral vector	1	-	March/April 2021	-	Phase III trial	Intramuscular

FDA, US Food and Drug Administration.

4. Sinovac
   - Aka Coronavac.
   - Developed by a Chinese biopharmaceutical company.
   - Clinical trials Phase I/II are randomized, double-blinded, and placebo controlled. A two-dose immunization is administered at a 28-day interval.
   - Inactivated vaccine.
   - Efficacy needs to be determined.
5. Bacillus Calmette-Guérin (BCG) (BRACE) trial
   - Murdoch children's Research Institute, Australia.
   - Suggested to have a role in protecting healthcare workers against the coronavirus disease.
   - Phase III, two-group, multicentric, randomized controlled trial.
   - BCG vaccine and 0.9% NaCl as placebo.
6. Sputnik V
   - The Gamaleya National Center of Epidemiology and Microbiology.
   - Two-vector vaccine against coronavirus.
   - An open, prospective, two-stage, non-randomized, first-phase study involving healthy volunteers.
   - Immunization is assessed at different points of duration by
     ◦ Antigen-specific antibody titer in blood serum by enzyme-linked immunosorbent assay (ELISA).
     ◦ Virus neutralizing antibody titer.
     ◦ Antigen-specific cellular immunity.
   - There is 92% efficacy.
7. Zydus (ZyCoV-D)
   - DNA vaccine
   - Phase I/II is an adaptive, multicentric, randomized, double-blind placebo-controlled trial that is ongoing.
8. Johnson & Johnson JNJ-78436725 (Ad26.COV2.S)
9. To assess the safety, reactogenicity, and immunogenicity of Ad26.COV2.S, which expresses the stabilized spike protein of SARS-CoV-2.
   - Safety profile and immunogenicity after a single dose warrants further study.
   - Phase 3 is a global study with 60,000 participants to determine safety and efficacy of single dose versus placebo in COVID presentations.

TABLE 10-2 COVID Vaccine-Related Adverse Effects

Vaccine	Adverse Events
Pfizer-BioNTech	• Local reactions (redness, swelling, pain at the injection site)
	• Systemic reactions (fever, headache, chills, vomiting, diarrhea, new or worsening muscle pain)
	• Lymphadenopathy
Moderna-mRNA-1273	• Local reactions (redness, swelling, pain at the injection site)
	• Systemic reaction (arthralgia, fatigue, fever, chills, headache, myalgia, nausea)
Oxford-AstraZeneca	• Common (arm pain, chills, fever, joint pains, muscle aches, fatigue, headache)
	• Uncommon (abdominal pain, hyperhidrosis, dizziness, decreased appetite, lymphadenopathy)
	• Special warning:
	› Thrombocytopenia and coagulation disorders (risk of bleeding/bruising)
	› Immunocompromised
Gamaleya (Sputnik V)	• Headache, fever, myalgias
Johnson & Johnson	• Fatigue, headache, myalgia, pain at the injection site, thromboembolic disease

COVID-19 CLINICAL RESEARCH

1. COVID19-0001-USR (Colombia)
   - Study to evaluate efficacy of COVID19-0001-USR in patients with mild/moderate COVID-19 infection in outpatients (COVID-19).
   - Randomized controlled, double-blind study with COVID19-0001-USR versus normal saline 3 mL self-administered via nebulization three times a day for 7 days (Table 10-2).
   - Estimated to start phases 1 and 2 on November 2, 2020.
   - Primary outcome measure is that the COVID19-0001-USR 1% nebulized pathway changes viral load of the SARS-CoV-2 virus (COVID-19) in the upper and lower airways if started during initial phase of infection.

2. COVID-19 convalescent plasma (CCP) transfusion
   - To evaluate the safety and clinical effectiveness of transfusing one unit of banked plasma obtained from patients who have recovered from the novel coronavirus SARS-CoV-2 infection with high titers of IgG antibody to this virus transfused into patients with high risk of progressing to severe coronavirus-induced disease (COVID-19).
   - Open label trial for severe COVID-19 infections (severity based on pulmonary infiltration, hypoxia, respiratory failure, sepsis, and multiple organ dysfunction, which is assessed by Sequential Organ Failure Assessment [SOFA] score).
   - Early phase 1 (start date: June 1, 2020; estimated completion date: May 31, 2021).
   - Primary outcome measures are to expect changes in pretransfusion respiratory status compared with day 3 respiratory status as measured by PaO_2/FiO_2 ratio, pulse oximetry, aO_2, respiratory rate, and intubation status.
   - Secondary outcome measures are to evaluate changes in SOFA scores, 8-point ordinal clinical deterioration scale, length of intensive care unit (ICU)/hospital stay, anti-CoV-2 IgM and IgG levels and be vigilant of presence of signs or symptoms of plasma transfusion reactions and/or immune complex disorders (as evidenced by fever spike, urticarial lesion, arthralgias, myalgias, hematuria, non-IgE-mediated anaphylaxis) at 1, 3, 7, and 28 days posttransfusion.
3. BTL-TML-COVID study
   - Study in adults (60+) to test effects of low-dose thimerosal on symptoms of COVID-19 and compare with placebo to show a difference in physical characteristics and viral levels.
   - In preclinical trials, BTL-TML interfered with translation of viral replication and structural integrity proteins of infected cells. Genomic studies have shown that BTL-TML downregulates several proinflammatory cytokine genes and upregulates anti-inflammatory genes.
   - Double-blind, placebo-controlled study, phase 2 trial (started on July 30, 2020 and estimated to be completed October 30, 2020).

- Primary outcome measure is the mean duration and severity of disease as assessed by change from baseline in the physical component summary of the Short Form-36 Quality of Life instrument 2 days post administration.
- Secondary outcome measure is to assess treatment-related adverse events (AEs), as gauged by the investigator as to severity, duration, and relationship to treatment for 2 weeks post administration.

4. Stanford Lambda study
   - Phase 2, open-label, single-blinded, randomized-controlled study of a single dose of peginterferon Lambda-1a compared with placebo in outpatients with mild COVID-19. Participants will be randomly assigned 1:1 to a single subcutaneous dose of Peginterferon Lambda-1a or placebo.
   - Interferons are a group of cytokines that have antiviral activity. Interferon lambda is a type III interferon that primarily works on epithelial cells in the respiratory tract, where SARS-CoV-2 replicates.
   - Interferon lambda inhibits viral replication without being proinflammatory.
   - Primary outcome was the duration of viral shedding in respiratory secretions in 28 days of follow-up, as measured by the time to the first of two consecutive negative respiratory secretions obtained by oropharyngeal and/or anterior nares swabs for SARS-CoV-2 by qRT-PCR (accomplished on August 14, 2020).
   - Secondary outcome measures include the SARS-CoV-2 viral load, area under the curve of SARS-CoV-2 viral load, time to alleviate all symptoms, and recording number of participants requiring hospitalization after 28 days.

5. SUNY Buffalo Melatonin Study
   - This study is a pilot randomized, double-blind, placebo-controlled clinical trial to evaluate the safety and efficacy of melatonin in adult outpatients suspected to be afflicted with COVID-19.
   - The study will aim to evaluate the clinical efficacy of 10 mg of melatonin compared with placebo as assessed by hospitalization, COVID-19–related symptoms, and mortality.

- Can the anti-inflammatory and antioxidant actions of melatonin reduce the severity and prevent progression of mild COVID-19?
- Phase 2: estimated start date is November 1, 2020, and estimated completion date is March 31, 2021.
- Primary outcome measures the cumulative incidence of treatment-emergent AEs. The study will evaluate the safety of the intervention through 28 days of follow-up compared with the control arm as assessed by cumulative incidence of serious adverse events (SAEs), cumulative incidence of grade 3 and 4 AEs, and/or discontinuation or temporary suspension of the investigational medication (for any reason).
- Secondary outcome measures include incidence of COVID–related hospitalization, COVID–related symptoms and mortality after 28 days, and rate of resolution of COVID–related symptoms assessed after 3, 7, 14, and 28 days.

6. Medical College of Wisconsin high-titer anti-SARS-CoV-2 plasma
   - Open-label, phase 2 study evaluating efficacy and safety of high-titer anti-SARS-CoV-2 convalescent donor plasma in an ICU versus non-ICU cohort study in hospitalized patients with acute severe respiratory symptoms from COVID.
   - Phase 2: start date was May 11, 2020 and estimated completion date is listed as May 1, 2023.
   - Primary outcome measures overall mortality within 60 days from infusion of plasma.
   - Secondary outcome measures length of ICU stay during current admission for COVID.

7. Tufts nitric oxide for preventing progression in COVID
   - Randomized-controlled (2:1) open-label investigation of inhaled nitric oxide (NO) to prevent progression to more advanced disease in 42 hospitalized patients with COVID-19, at risk for worsening, based on baseline systemic oxygenation and two or more of the major risk factors of age >60 years, type II diabetes mellitus, hypertension, and obesity.
   - Phase 2: start date was May 12, 2020 and estimated completion date is listed as July 31, 2021.

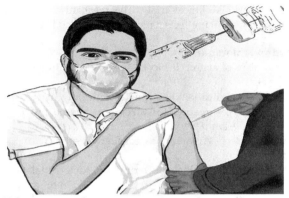

FIGURE 10-2 Demonstration of COVID vaccine.

- Primary outcome was the prevention of progressive systemic de-oxygenation, with escalation to higher levels of oxygen and ventilatory support or death, assessed using a 7-point severity scale over the course of 28 days.
- Secondary outcome measures include prevention of progression assessed by alternative severity scale, time to reach maximal severity scale, proportion of patients in each stage at maximum severity, PaO_2/FiO_2 or SaO_2/FiO_2 ratio, measured daily, length of hospital stay, frequency of intubation, extracorporeal membrane oxygenation (ECMO), or need to intubate with a do-not-resuscitate order (DNR) and mortality after 28 days.
- Secondary outcome also measures interleukin (IL)-6, tumor necrosis factor (TNF)-α, fibrinogen, C-reactive protein, ferritin, and D-dimer levels over a course of 7 days (Figure 10-2).

COVID-19 MEDICATION AND CARDIOVASCULAR EFFECTS

The management of COVID-19 consists of infection prevention, case detection, and monitoring along with supportive care. The following medications have been used in treatment of COVID-19 infected patients in various clinical trials. The mechanism of action and adverse cardiovascular effects have been discussed here.

- **Hydroxychloroquine**

  Mechanism of action: It blocks Toll-like receptors on dendritic cells.

  Role: This medication, along with azithromycin, was used for COVID-19 treatment. Currently it has no proven role in COVID-19 infection.

  Adverse effects: Arrhythmias, cardiomyopathy.

- **Azithromycin**

  Mechanism of action: Bacteriostatic/bactericidal (binds to 50S ribosomal subunit, inhibit protein synthesis), activity against proinflammatory cytokines (IL-6 and IL-8), and prevention of cytokine storm (experimental role).

  Adverse effects: Prolonged QTc and it has drug-drug interactions.

- **Dexamethasone**

  Mechanism of action: Inhibits multiple inflammatory cytokines, and produces multiple glucocorticoid and mineralocorticoid effects.

  Role: It has been widely used for the treatment of severe acute respiratory syndrome (SARS), Middle East respiratory syndrome (MERS), influenza, and pneumonia. It is an essential medication on WHO's list of medications for COVID-19 management.

  Adverse effects: Hypertension and heart failure exacerbation.

- **Ibuprofen**

  Mechanism of action: Inhibits cyclooxygenase, reducing prostaglandins.

  Concern: In France, the medication is believed to upregulate the expression of the angiotensin-converting enzyme 2 (ACE2) receptor, which is believed to be the mode of entry for SARS-CoV-2. This resulted in decreased use of this medication.

- **Remdesivir**

  Mechanism of action: Inhibits RNA-dependent RNA polymerase, prevents viral replication.

Role: Remdesivir has shown benefit in reducing the severity of COVID-19–related respiratory illness.

Adverse effects: Sinus bradycardia and prolonged QTc.

- **Convalescent Plasma**

  Mechanism of action: Unclear. A possible explanation is that the antibodies from the plasma of a recovered patient results in the suppression of the viremia.

  Role: In 2014 during the Ebola outbreak, WHO recommended the use of convalescent plasma from recovered patients as empirical treatment during outbreaks. Improved rates of nasopharyngeal viral clearance are seen in severe COVID-19.

- **Lopinavir/ritonavir**

  Mechanism of action: Protease inhibitors; no clinical benefits (still investigational).

  Adverse effect: Hyperlipidemia.

- **Tocilizumab**

  Mechanism of action: Humanized monoclonal antibody against the IL-6 receptor (experimental role).

- **Bamlanivimab**

  Mechanism of action: It binds to the receptor binding domain of the spike protein of SARS-CoV-2, blocking the spike protein's attachment to the human ACE2 receptor.

  Adverse effects: No known cardiovascular reactions.

COVID-19 MEDICATION INTERACTIONS WITH CARDIAC MEDICTION

COVID-19 infection in patients with cardiovascular diseases have been discussed in this book. There have been considerable reports of AEs secondary to drug-drug interactions between COVID-19 medications and certain cardiac medications. Table 10-3 represents the drug-drug interactions.

TABLE 10-3 Medications Interactions with COVID Treatment

Cardiovascular Medication/Class	Lopinavir/Ritonavir	Bamlanivimab	Remdesivir	Tocilizumab
Antiarrhythmics				
Amiodarone	Increase	Neutral	Neutral	Neutral
Dofetilide	Increase	Neutral	Neutral	Neutral
Flecainide	Increase	Neutral	Neutral	Neutral
Mexiletine	Increase	Neutral	Neutral	Neutral
Propafenone	Increase	Neutral	Neutral	Neutral
Anticoagulants				
Apixaban	Increase	Neutral	Neutral	Decrease
Dabigatran	Neutral/Decrease	Neutral	Neutral	Neutral
Edoxaban	Increase	Neutral	Neutral	Neutral
Enoxaparin	Neutral	Neutral	Neutral	Neutral
Heparin	Neutral	Neutral	Neutral	Neutral
Rivaroxaban	Increase	Neutral	Neutral	Decrease
Warfarin	Increase/Decrease	Neutral	Neutral	Decrease
Antihypertensives				
Beta blockers	Increase	Neutral	Neutral	Neutral
Diltiazem/verapamil	Increase	Neutral	Neutral	Neutral
Amlodipine	Increase	Neutral	Neutral	Neutral
Epleronone		Neutral	Neutral	Neutral
Fosinopril	Increase	Neutral	Neutral	Neutral
Irbesartan/losartan	Decrease	Neutral	Neutral	Neutral
Spironolactone	Neutral	Neutral	Neutral	Neutral
Sacubitril/valsartan	Increase	Neutral	Neutral	Neutral
Valsartan	Increase	Neutral	Neutral	Neutral

(*Continued*)

TABLE 10-3 Medications Interactions with COVID Treatment (*Continued*)

Cardiovascular Medication/Class	Lopinavir/Ritonavir	Bamlanivimab	Remdesivir	Tocilizumab
Antiplatelets				
Aspirin	Neutral	Neutral	Neutral	Neutral
Clopidogrel	Decrease	Neutral	Neutral	Decrease
Prasugrel	Neutral	Neutral	Neutral	Decrease
Ticagrelor	Increase	Neutral	Neutral	Decrease
Lipid-Lowering Therapies				
Atorvastatin	Increase max: 20 mg	Neutral	Neutral	Decrease
Ezetimibe	Neutral	Neutral	Neutral	Neutral
Fenofibrates	Neutral	Neutral	Neutral	Neutral
Fluvastatin	Neutral	Neutral	Neutral	Decrease
Gemfibrozil	Decrease	Neutral	Neutral	Neutral
Lovastatin	Increase	Neutral	Neutral	Decrease
Pitavastatin	Neutral	Neutral	Neutral	Neutral
Pravastatin	Neutral	Neutral	Neutral	Neutral
Rosuvastatin	Increase max: 20 mg	Neutral	Neutral	Decrease
Simvastatin	Neutral	Neutral	Neutral	Decrease
Other				
Digoxin	Increase	unknown	Neutral	Neutral
Ivabradine	Increase	Neutral	Neutral	Neutral
Ranolazine	Increase	Neutral	Neutral	Neutral

REMOTE MONITORING

Several strategies to prevent outbreak of COVID-19 infection have been proposed. Minimizing clinic visits, especially in immunocompromised patients, is suggested by use of telehealth visits. Many patients fear that they will be exposed to COVID-19 from their visit to a healthcare facility. The healthcare system had to rapidly evolve and come up with alternatives to provide adequate health-care services without exposing patients to the virus. It is crucial to understand that there is no single FDA-approved measure or device, but the FDA is trying to fast-track approvals for COVID-19–related remote monitoring. (1-2)

- Telemedicine: Zoom, FaceTime, WhatsApp.
- Kardia 61 remote monitoring ECG device: AliveCor has been working on an algorithm for fast-tracking QT screening.
- Multiple smartwatches: Apple Watch and Fitbit are being used in various studies to report vitals and real-time surveillance of contagious viral illness. Various digital technology companies are working on using the data from these watches to help con-tact trace COVID-positive patients.
- NYC Test & Trace Corps: Community support system for those who tested positive that provides a wide range of services depending on the severity of the symptoms, such as medication delivery, free hotel room for isolation purposes, and frequent check-ins with the patient (Figure 10-3).

KEY POINTS

- COVID-19 vaccine may have a role in preventing the spread of infection, but long-term effects are unknown.
- There have been many investigational drugs that may have a potential benefit in the management of COVID-19 infection.

PATIENT EDUCATION

Is the COVID-19 vaccine effective?
Clinical trials have shown that the COVID-19 vaccine is 95% effec-tive in preventing COVID-19 infection. It consists of two doses of intramuscular injections given almost 4 weeks apart.
What are the adverse effects of the vaccine?
Rash, headache, and myalgia are common after the second dose of vaccine. The symptoms usually last for 24-48 hours. If symp-toms persist after 48 hours, medical attention should be sought.

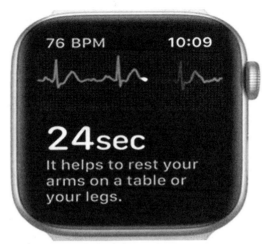

FIGURE 10-3 Cardiac remote monitoring device.

Do I still wear mask after vaccine?

Social distancing and face mask should be practiced even after vaccine to prevent the spread of virus.

Do I need a vaccine if I get COVID-19 infection?

The antibody titers can wane with time. People who suffered from COVID-19 should also receive the COVID vaccine to boost immunity against the infection.

References

1. UPDATED Comparing COVID-19 Vaccines: Timelines, Types and Prices | BioSpace
2. Vaccine clinical comparison (vizientinc.com)

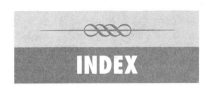

INDEX

Note: Page numbers followed by *f* and *t* represent figures and tables, respectively.